Hospital English
the *Brilliant* learning workbook for international nurses

Catharine Arakelian

Mark Bartram

Alison Magnall

Radcliffe Medical Press

Radcliffe Medical Press Ltd
18 Marcham Road
Abingdon
Oxon OX14 1AA
United Kingdom

www.radcliffe-oxford.com
The Radcliffe Medical Press electronic catalogue and online ordering facility.
Direct sales to anywhere in the world.

Hospital English: the brilliant learning workbook for international nurses

British Library Cataloguing in Publication Data

A catalogue record for this book is available from the British Library.

ISBN 1 85775 864 1

Typeset by Meg Richardson
Printed and bound by T J International, Padstow, Cornwall

Contents

Hospital English – *Brilliant* summary of the units

Unit	Professional Focus	Working with Others	Language Study	Scope of Practice	Assignment
1	The National Health Service	If you don't know, ask Where I work	Noticing 'real'English Words words words Cultural map of chatting	The pluses and minuses of working in the UK	Make a detailed plan of your clinical area
2	Who do you know?	Taking phone calls	Hello Goodbye Words that stand out	Organisation of care	Make an organisation chart of all the people who work in your clinical area
3	Admitting your patient	Maria's story - Asking your supervisor for feedback	Intonation's important, innit? What use is a dictionary? Sub-technical language	Kolb and reflective learning	Create a user guide for a piece of equipment
4	Confidentiality	How's your bridging?	Short forms Linking sounds together Telling an anecdote	Acknowledging your limitations	Make a profile of one patient's experience of hospital
5	Health promotion	Handover	Hospital diet lexicon Making suggestions Rhythm of English	Interpreting graphs	Prepare a short talk on a clinical subject
6	Moving and handling	Communication while moving a patient Maria's story - Assertiveness	Moving and handling lexicon Word families	Being part of a team The ward round	Interview two members of your team. Make a questionnaire
7	Transfering your patient	Making phone calls	Record keeping	The legal framework	Transfer of care in your hospital
8	Infection control	Communication while giving personal care	Did you get a sample? Slang on the loo Present your talk	Your competency framework	Assess your language and communication skills and make an action plan

Acknowledgements

The programme is indebted to the five hundred plus international nurses from twenty-three different countries who have worked and studied with us over the last four years at the Oxford Radcliffe Hospitals NHS Trust, the University Hospitals of Leicester NHS Trust and other hospitals. They have tested our new ideas, suggested improvements and shown honesty, courage and a sense of humour throughout. We are particularly grateful to the international nurses who commented on the first drafts of this book.

Units 1-4 were originally published by Arakelian as *Hospital English: The Essential Communication Programme for International Nurses Book 1.*

The authors would like to thank all the lecturers at Oxford Brookes University who contributed their ideas to the programmes delivered in 1999–2001.

A big thank you to the current Arakelian licensed associate teachers: Sally Ballard, Christine Dowling, Stephanie Gosling, Juliet Henderson, Ann Lee, Mark O' Rourke, Carole Robinson, Lyndsey Senior, George Taylor and Felicity Ziegler who continue to improve the teaching and learning experience with their nurses and in the process improve our understanding of what it feels like to settle and work in a new culture.

A particular thank you is owed to Marion Pahlen, now teaching in Germany, for her generous contribution of the ideas behind giving and getting feedback.

Thank you to our families who have allowed us the space to write.

Foreword

by Maura Buchanan BA RGN
PGDip (Clinical Neurosciences)

Deputy President,
Royal College of Nursing
Senior Nurse,
Oxford Radcliffe Hospitals NHS Trust.

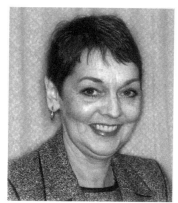

Communicating effectively in a foreign language requires a level of understanding that goes far beyond the learning of vocabulary and grammar.

Textbook English is seldom the language of the workplace. Apparently familiar words and phrases may both amuse and confuse the learner when used in different contexts. Nowhere is this more evident than in the field of healthcare.

The Arakelian Programme introduces international nurses to the culture of the health service in the United Kingdom.

Catharine Arakelian has demonstrated tremendous insight into the development of communication and language skills. Her approach makes learning English a fun experience. The exercises encourage good listening and observation skills, essential elements of mastering a foreign language.

Many international nurses have already completed the programme and have successfully adapted to our health service, including some working with me in Oxford. It has been a joy to see their communication skills develop as the programme progresses. Their confidence and their professionalism are testimony to the success of this approach.

This book will serve as a useful tool for mentors and supervisors of international nurses. Mentors will gain greater self-awareness and some insight into the peculiarities of our own culture.

Nursing is a truly global profession, providing opportunities for individuals to gain valuable experience in other healthcare systems. International nurses have much to offer us. Their own cultures, as well as their clinical skills, greatly enrich UK nursing.

In today's multicultural health service, good communication is key to safe nursing practice and to the delivery of a service that meets the needs of patients, similarly from diverse backgrounds. I am sure that this series of books will provide a solid foundation enabling international nurses to competently practise their profession in the UK.

Maura Buchanan

About the authors

Catharine Arakelian, BA RSA Dip TEFLA

Catharine is an intercultural education consultant, teacher trainer and researcher in adult migrant worker education. She graduated from Bristol University in 1984 and worked as a theatre director. Between 1994-2001 she was a senior lecturer at Oxford Brookes University where she was Director of the Oxford Brookes University International Summer School.

Mark Bartram, BA RSA Dip TEFLA

Mark is an English Language Teaching consultant, writer and teacher trainer. He graduated from Durham University in 1979, before going to live and work in Italy. On coming back to the UK in 1989, he was the academic director of a language school in Oxford for 10 years before setting up Atlas English, an English language school for juniors. He has published numerous books on English language teaching, including Correction (LTP) and Initiative (CUP).

Alison Magnall, MA RSA Cert TEFLA RN RSCN HVCert

Alison qualified as a general and paediatric nurse in 1985 at Alder Hey. She worked as a Health Visitor for six years in London. She maintained her registration and continued working after completing her degree at the University of Oxford. Since 1999 she has worked with international nurses on Arakelian Programmes developing specialist teaching materials and co-writing Hospital English.

To the International Nurse

Welcome!

It's *Brilliant* to see you!

You are an expert in your field.

You have had many years of training and experience.

You are needed and welcome.

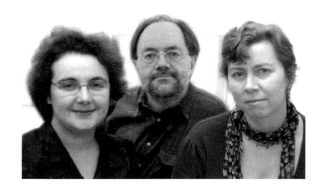

Whether you have been here for a few months or have just arrived, this working environment is still very new to you. Adjusting to the working culture of the UK will take you some time. Don't be surprised!

This short programme in communication skills gives you new confidence to make the changes and to equip you with some personal survival strategies so you can work, study and live without becoming over-stressed.

In fact, we want you to feel *Brilliant!*

Your career in the UK has no ceiling. You can be the best and earn the best if you believe in your own power and potential. This programme will show you how to turn your aspirations into realities by working with others as a valued professional.

Welcome and good luck in your new jobs. Be *Brilliant!*

Catharine Arakelian   Mark Bartram   Alison Magnall

How to use this book

This book is for you to use by yourself in the hospital where you work or in a classroom with a trainer or language teacher.

If you are working through this book by yourself, talk to your supervisors about the tasks and find someone, preferably a native speaker or someone who has been in the UK for several years, who will act as a mentor. You should write your answers in the book and show them to others so you can practise your new skills with your team and the other people around you. Normally you will find that people are very interested in your workbook and will want to help you.

It is more effective (and much more fun) to follow this workbook with a friend. Try to find another nurse in the hospital who might want to work alongside you on this course.

See Working with a *Brilliant* Buddy on page 167.

How this book is organised

There are eight units which provide around three hours structured study each week and many opportunities for reflection and observation in the workplace.

Each unit has four sections:

 Language Study

We find out why English can seem so hard to hear and how you can be more easily heard by your team and patients. We look at how native speakers speak so fast and how to improve your own listening skills.

 Professional Focus

We look at aspects of your duties in an acute hospital from handover to discharge planning. We look at how you communicate with your team and your patients – what words you say and how you say them.

Remember every hospital has its own policies and procedures so we invite you to check all the information with a more senior team member to see how it is the same or how it is different from your previous workplace.

 Working with Others

This section shows you how to become recognised as a good team-player and communicator by adopting culturally appropriate strategies that really work. We show you how to be effective in common workplace situations such as giving and receiving feedback on your work.

👁 Understanding your Scope of Practice

Better communication skills and greater confidence lead to more opportunities for taking on responsibilities and extending your professional role. This section looks in detail at aspects of the United Kingdom Nursing and Midwifery Council Code of Professional Conduct and helps you understand what is meant by such terms as accountability and autonomy.

Exercises, tasks and assignments

Complete these tasks either in class or in your own time when you are at work.

Some exercises provide quick practice in aspects of language – normally vocabulary and pronunciation. (If you feel you need more language development then you may need to go to a bookshop and buy a good grammar practice book in General English.)

Tasks are either **observation** or **reflective** tasks.

Observation tasks need to be carried out while you are at work. They build up your understanding of the behaviour and language around you.

Reflective tasks can be carried out while you are on the bus or in a quiet corner. These aim to bring together your knowledge and experience so you can grow in self-awareness and plan your own learning.

✎ There is an **assignment** at the end of each unit. This is a more substantial piece of work which you can start keeping in your *Brilliant* portfolio.

See Building My *Brilliant* Portfolio on p 166.

🔑 Answer keys to exercises

The answers to a number of the exercises are at the back of the book. Look out for the key symbol. These are suggested answers only. Your answers may be equally as good. Try to answer the questions from your own experience before turning to the key.

References

References are written in the text next to the quotation. Most of the books and journals in the references should be available in your hospital library.

You might decide that you don't need to do every assignment and task. That's fine! You can dip in and do any task or exercise in any order if you want. Do what you have time and energy for.

Your new professional identity

Adapting to a new workplace requires an effort to build the professional identity you wish to project. You have to balance the need to earn the trust of your colleagues because you are an unknown quantity, against losing face by revealing your own lack of knowledge of the new workplace.

You need to find a professional way of demonstrating and sharing your clinical expertise within the legal framework of the UK whilst clearly expressing your own needs. Your team and supervisor will help you to learn.

You can help them by writing about your progress and being honest about your experience – the ups and downs. We teach you how to create and use two special books – My Professional Identity Notebook and My Personal Lexicon – for these notes. Your communication skills will quickly improve and you can use these to reinforce your value and skills in the hospital.

Your cultural map

The knowledge about how to behave in a certain situation can be considered metaphorically as a behaviour map which is culturally accurate.

Your old behaviour map, which perfectly fits your previous culture, may not be useful in predicting how your actions will be viewed in the new culture.

Your behaviour may not have the desired effect. Other people may see you as rude or passive. They may simply avoid trying to understand you by referring to their own cultural map of prejudice to explain your behaviour.

As you work through this book you will be building up knowledge about how people behave in this culture. The book and the people around you, if you ask them, will guide you. This knowledge constitutes a new cultural map which you can now use to develop your relationships and nursing practice.

You may need to change your own behaviour so do not expect results immediately. You will certainly need to practise new culturally appropriate behaviours before they seem natural to you. Remember your cultural map may not be complete and you may need additional experiences before it is consistently useful.

As a competent international nurse you will have been making these maps throughout your travels. On this programme we make the process explicit so you can explore and develop quickly in a safe environment.

There are cultural maps specific to the NHS, and even more subtle ones specific to your own hospital and clinical area. You will develop your noticing skills on this programme and will soon have mapped the uncharted territories! All this work we ask you to keep in My Professional Identity Notebook. After that, it is up to you!

Stages on the journey of cultural adaptation

Cultural Adjustment Curve

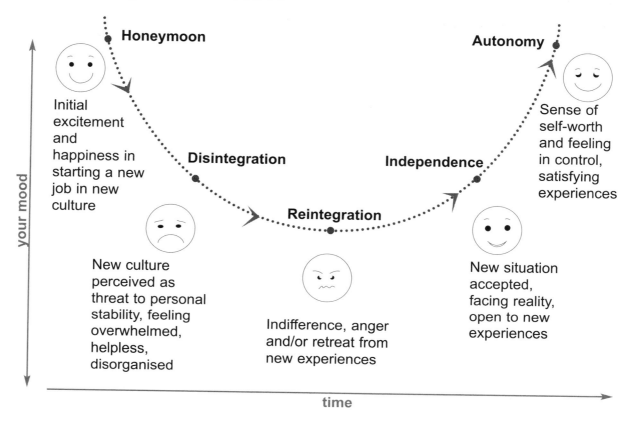

Cultural adaptation

In adapting to a new culture you go through different stages of emotional adjustment. The stages are called honeymoon, disintegration, reintegration, independence and autonomy. You may be in the honeymoon stage for a long time if you have a well-supported induction programme.

You don't necessarily spend very long at each stage and you probably don't spend an equal amount of time at each stage. You may not even be conscious of the different stages but when you look back on your first year in a new culture you might be able to identify when you moved through each stage. The crucial thing is not to get stuck in the negative stages. When you experience the lows, recognise that they are a normal part of adjusting to a new culture and relax. You may find that being able to identify where you are on your psychological journey helps you feel better and move on.

It is quite normal for this adjustment process to take a year or more before you feel really comfortable in your new cultural shoes.

Are you feeling well adjusted?

Consider the Cultural Adjustment Curve on page 13 which describes what you might be going through in each stage.

Over the next few months mark your current mood on the chart. Every week record your new level of confidence. Time is marked along the horizontal axis (measured in weeks). The vertical axis is indicating your confidence and so could be said to be measuring your 'adjustment'. I hope you have an ever rising curve!

You may find that if you are transferred to a new area or move to a new role or take on new responsibilities you go through the same stages all over again but now perhaps you can recognise the cycle and cope better.

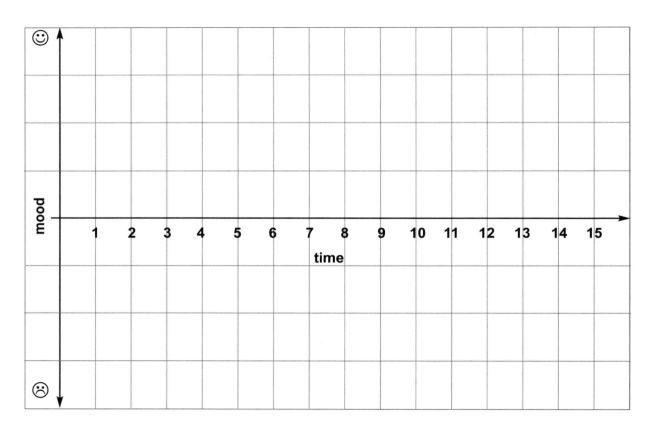

Remember it's natural to feel out of your depth when you're out of your culture but you'll soon be getting along swimmingly

Getting ready

You will need

Essential

- Hospital English: the *Brilliant* learning workbook for international nurses
- Pen or pencil
- Energy

Useful

- **My Personal Lexicon**

  Please buy an A5 or smaller bound notebook to be My Personal Lexicon

  A lexicon is a collection of words. My Personal Lexicon – your own personal collection of words – you can build up when talking with your patients, colleagues and friends. Note down new words you hear in the workplace as you find them – ask for explanations if they are unfamiliar to you.

- **My Professional Identity Notebook**

  Please buy an A5 or A4 bound notebook to be My Professional Identity Notebook.

  Reflective practice enables you to learn effectively from your work and personal experience. Throughout the programme you are invited to note critical incidents in your professional and social life and to reflect on your experiences.

Desirable

- A *Brilliant* Buddy – See page 167

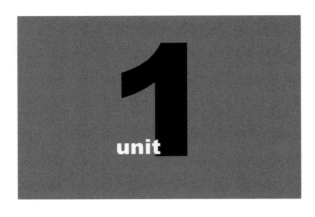

 Noticing 'real' English
Words words words
Cultural map of chatting

 If you don't know, ask
Where I work

 The National Health Service

 The pluses and minuses of working
in the UK

 Make a detailed plan of your
clinical area

1.1 Noticing 'real' English

Even if you have studied the English language for a long time, you may find the 'real' English you hear every day in the UK is very different!

'Real' English

- is spoken very quickly
- uses different or unusual expressions – and even different grammar.

1.1.a

 Look at the six expressions below and decide if they were said by
- **a nurse (N)**
- **a patient (P) or**
- **a friend outside work (F).**

Mark them with N, P or F accordingly. Some of them may have more than one answer! There is an example to help you.

1	*That's healing up nicely.*	N
2	*Fancy a drink this evening?*	......
3	*Just pop your foot up here.*	......
4	*I'm getting a lot of sharp pains up the side.*	......
5	*This is the offending ankle, is it?*	......
6	*It just doesn't seem to have come right.*	......
7	*What did you get up to at the weekend?*	......

What did you notice about these expressions? One thing is that we often miss out words – for example '*(Do you) fancy a drink this evening?*' in example 1.1.a 2. Second, we often use slang or colloquial words instead of the 'proper' ones – e.g. *pop* instead of *place* or *put* in example 1.1.a 3 or *get up to* in example 1.1.a 7.

Finally we can use ironic or slightly jokey language to reassure the patient, or to make a bond with the patient, as in *the offending ankle* in example 1.1.a 5.

Word partnerships

1.1.b

 Match the verb on the left with the phrase on the right to make useful expressions. The first one has been done for you.

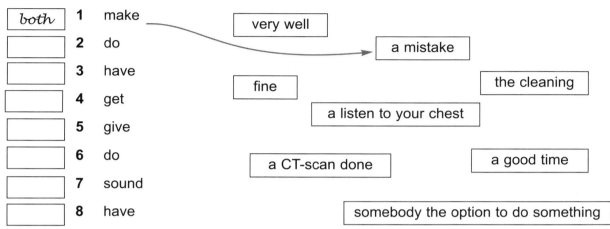

both	**1**	make
	2	do
	3	have
	4	get
	5	give
	6	do
	7	sound
	8	have

very well

a mistake

fine

the cleaning

a listen to your chest

a CT-scan done

a good time

somebody the option to do something

These expressions are very common in spoken English. You will find it is much easier to talk to colleagues and patients (and understand them) if you can use word partnerships like these.

1.1.c

Label the word partnerships above according to where you would hear them. Which ones in the task above would be used:

- **in everyday English conversation outside work (EE)**
- **on the ward – Hospital English (HE)**
- **both?**

The first one has been done for you.

1.1.d

Collect six word partnerships, three from outside work, and three from the ward. Write them in the box below:

Buy a spiral bound notebook that will fit in your pocket and start writing down useful word partnerships and expressions you hear. Call this book My Personal Lexicon

17

1.2 Words words words

One of the most useful tools you can have to improve your communication is a small notebook in which to write down useful words and expressions that you notice around you. Call this notebook My Personal Lexicon.

1.2.a

Here is a quiz about My Personal Lexicon. For each question, only one answer is correct. See how many you can get right!

1 How big should a lexicon be?

a too big for your pocket
b just big enough to fit in your pocket
c so small you can lose it easily

b

2 Why should I write new words and expressions down?

a so that I can forget about them
b to waste a bit of time at work
c to remember them more easily

3 Should I organise the lexicon in some way?

a yes, that makes it easier to find things
b no, better to have it a complete mess
c it doesn't matter as long as you're happy

4 What things should I write down?

a anything that you might find useful in the future
b everything you can
c as little as possible

5 Should I write down abbreviations like DNA*?

a no, you'll be using them every day, so there's no need
b yes, any and every abbreviation will be useful
c it's up to you
   * if you don't know what this means, ask!

6 If I notice a new word, how should I write it down?

a on its own, then you won't get confused
b in an expression or chunk
c with words that start with the same letter

7 What else should I write down about the word?

a nothing, you haven't got room in a small book
b everything you can
c anything important or useful about it

8 What do you mean by important or useful?

a spelling
b pronunciation
c style (if the word is very formal or slang)
d technical or non-technical
e if it's British or American English
f any or all of the above if you think they are important

9. What other use is there for My Personal Lexicon?

a to write notes for your blockbusting novel about hospital life
b to make shopping lists
c to use as a tool for communication

10 What do you mean by a 'tool for communication'?

a because if your colleagues see you are writing things down, they will be more helpful, speak slower etc
b because if you write things down, you'll remember more and so speak better
c because if your colleagues see you writing, they'll think you really want to learn, and so they will be more willing to communicate with you

Don't forget to tell people what you are doing otherwise they may feel you are spying on them! Try saying

- That's interesting. Do you mind if I write that down? or

- I'd like to write that down. Is that okay? How do you spell that?

Wajagunnadooabahdit?

English people speak so quickly!
Have you noticed this?

You might hear a person say $\quad$ *kappatee?*

and it takes you five seconds to realise they were saying $\quad$ *A cup of tea?*
by which time they have gone off somewhere and
you've lost a chance to have a drink!

Or they might say $\quad$ *wajagunnadooabahdit?*

and you only understand later that they were saying $\quad$ *What are you going to do about it?*

The English do speak quickly: *kappatee* sounds like one word, but in fact it is 4! But that is not the only reason they are difficult to understand. A second reason is that English people do not say all the sounds equally, and in fact they pronounce certain sounds very quickly and 'weakly'. This is why people often say the English 'eat' their words.

More examples:

How would you say this word: *America.* Try asking an English person to say it. They will probably say something like

uh – mair – ri – kuh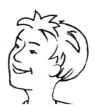

and the quicker they say it, the more they sound like they are eating the word.

Now try these words:

> *banana* $\qquad$ *photograph* $\qquad$ *policeman*

You can hear that one or two parts of the words are said much more strongly or loudly than the others:

> *aMERica,* $\quad$ *baNANa,* $\qquad$ *PHOtograph,* $\quad$ *poLICEman.*

The other bits get lost, or eaten. We say that the strong bits are **stressed** and the 'eaten' bits are **unstressed**.

1.2.b

Look at these six words from clinical settings. Indicate the bit of the word which is stressed (said most strongly).

radiographer	*intravenous*
condition	*deteriorate*
haemorrhage	*department*

It is not only true of words. The same thing happens with expressions and whole sentences. Look at this common expression: *Nice to meet you.*

Ask an English colleague to say it naturally. Which bit is stressed?
Most people stress the word *meet*:

> *Nice to MEET you.*

> o o O o
(Or, with bubbles: *Nice to meet you.*)

If you get the stressed bit right, it often doesn't matter much how you pronounce the other bits. And when you listen, listen out for the stressed bit, as that is the important bit.

1.2.c

Look at these common expressions. Mark the bit which is stressed. The first one is done for you.

O
1 Please sit down.

2 Have a nice day!

3 Mutton dressed as lamb.

4 Who's a mucky pup?

5 What did your last servant die of?

Do you know when we use these expressions? Find out from a colleague!

1.3 Cultural map of chatting

1.3.a

Are these statements usually true or false
a   about Britain
b   about your country?
Write T or F in the box

	Britain	Your country
It is normal to start a conversation by talking about the traffic.	☐	☐
People at parties will introduce themselves without being introduced by the host.	☐	☐
It is perfectly OK to chat socially to a patient you do not know.	☐	☐
If a woman is invited out for a drink by a man, it is perfectly OK to say no.	☐	☐
You do not ask for someone's telephone number the first time you meet.	☐	☐
It is OK to be a little late for a dinner party, but if you are very late, you must apologise.	☐	☐
Vegetarians are seen as very strange people.	☐	☐

1.3.b

Have you noticed what British people say when they are chatting?
Write down what they say:

to introduce the topic of the weather

Bit chilly today, isn't it?

to introduce themselves informally

to ask for someone's telephone number

to refuse an invitation

to apologise for being late

21

Chatting about youself

As an international nurse, many people will be interested in you and your background.

So you will often need to pass over information about yourself in a brief and interesting way. This will help other people to:

- engage with you
- remember you afterwards!

One way is to develop a quick chatty biography about yourself.

This should include:

name *I'm* ....

country of origin *I'm from* ....

what you are hoping to do in the UK (future plans)

I'm looking forward to ....

an open question which helps to make a bridge
to the other person

What about you ....

If your name is particularly interesting, you could say something about that.

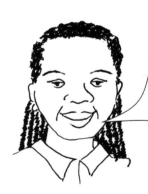

Hi - My name is Sentebaleng, I've just started on Ward 4 — I come from South Africa. My name means Forget-me-not. I'm just getting to know about UK names. Do any English names have meanings?

Hi — I'm Lani from the Philippines. I'm new to Ward 4 but I'm looking forward to having my own patients soon. It's a really big hospital. What do you think I should get to know first about working here? How do you think I could get to know the people here better?

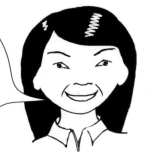

22

1.3.c

Try and do the same thing for yourself. What would you say? Write some notes in the bubble and then use the notes to make a quick biography about yourself.

Choose a quiet place where you won't be disturbed, such as your bathroom. Practise your spiel on your own. Then try it out on a colleague and see what they think. After you are happy with it, go out and try it on everybody you meet socially. The more you try it, the better it will sound.

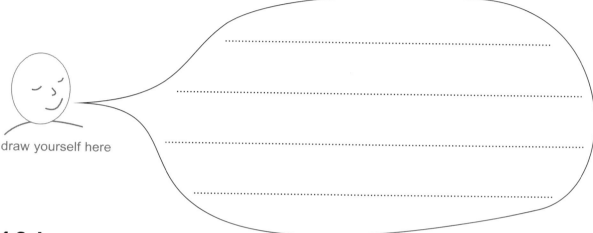

draw yourself here

1.3.d

People are interested in why so many international nurses are working in the UK. Answer these common questions in a brief but polite way.

You don't need to give your whole life story but it's good to have a short answer that you are comfortable with.

Why did you come to work in this hospital? **Why did you come to work in the UK?**

1.4   If you don't know, ask

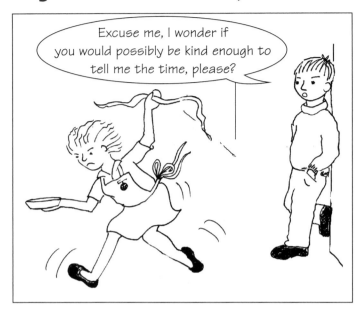

In the modern world, everybody needs information. Whether we are new to a job, have just come on shift, or simply have never been told, we need to know.

1.4.a

Think of some information you would like to know. Write it as a question or request here.

Look at the flow-chart
Work through the flow-chart for that particular request.
Now go out and get the answer to your question!

How to ask if you don't know

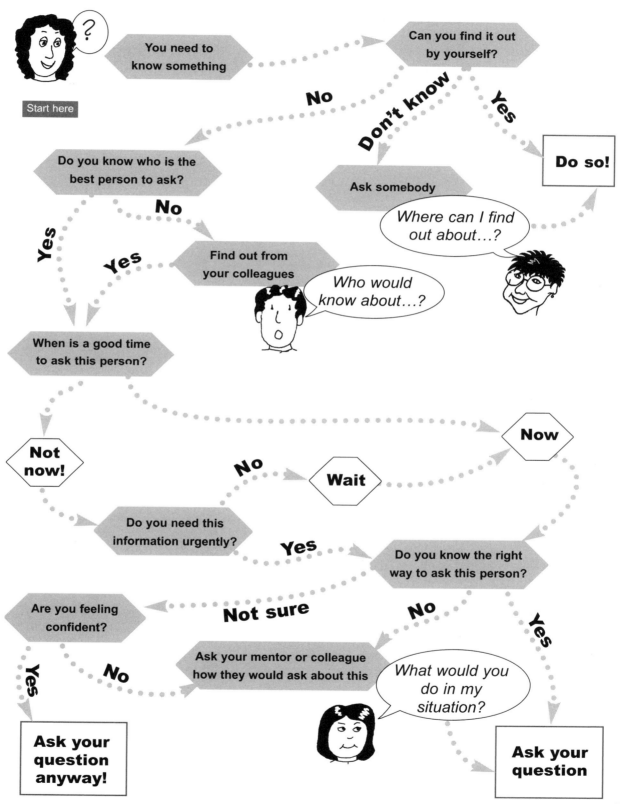

Start here

You need to know something

Can you find it out by yourself?

No

Don't know

Yes

Do so!

Do you know who is the best person to ask?

Ask somebody

Where can I find out about…?

No

Yes

Yes

Find out from your colleagues

Who would know about…?

When is a good time to ask this person?

Not now!

Now

No

Wait

Do you need this information urgently?

Yes

Do you know the right way to ask this person?

Are you feeling confident?

Not sure

No

Yes

Ask your mentor or colleague how they would ask about this

What would you do in my situation?

Yes

No

Ask your question anyway!

Ask your question

1.4.b

Make a list of information questions you hear asked by others on the ward. Write them in the box below.

Agree a good time with your supervisor. Explain to your colleagues that you are about to take a short time to observe and take notes.

The nurse's station might be a good place to observe requests being made.

Questions I heard today

1.4.c

Complete the table.

You need to know …	Who do you ask?	What do you say?
when a patient was admitted		
where the new (blank) drug charts are kept		
if you can take a study day off next week		
if a patient has been refusing their medication on the previous shift		
what the expression 'sick as a parrot' means		
your supervisor's contact telephone number		

1.5 Where I work

You need to be able to describe quickly and confidently where you work for visitors to the hospital and on social occasions.

1.5.a

Describe to a friend the place where you work by filling in the following and deleting what is not relevant.

> Go down the corridor. Take the lift to the second floor. As you come out of the lift, turn left, go through the green door and the X-ray department is on the right

I'm a nurse at...Hospital

I'm on the ....ward/in the .... department

Most of my patients are being treated for ....

We look after people with.../...

1.5.b

Give directions to a patient's relative how to reach your area from the main entrance of the hospital.

Give directions to a patient's relative how to get to your hospital.

What bus would they need to catch to get to the hospital? Is there a charge for parking? Are there visitors' hours?

1.6 The National Health Service

As an international nurse working in the United Kingdom here are a few facts you should know about the National Health Service. The NHS was founded in 1948 to provide free medical advice and treatment for anyone who needed it. The service was paid for primarily out of central taxes. The services before this date would vary across the country and according to the amount you could afford to pay.

When people feel sick they go first to their doctor, also known as their GP. GP stands for General Practitioner. A visit to the GP is free and prescriptions are free to many people. The GP might refer you to a hospital consultant.

A visit to a NHS hospital is free and the medicines given in hospital are free.

All necessary surgical treatment in an NHS hospital is free (but you might need to wait).

Over fifty years later many of the founding principles still apply. Throughout the late 1980s and 1990s a number of changes were brought about. The reasons for this were that:

- the cost of running the NHS was escalating
- the cost of treatment was rising in part due to advances in medical sciences
- public expectations were rising leading people to demand treatment as quickly as possible
- the UK has an increasingly ageing population.

This means that the NHS is going through a process of change which is not always easy to understand or to manage.

Policies and initiatives you might like to look at are

- The Health Act of 1999 which required NHS organisations to account for the quality of their services
- The NHS Plan (2000) which was introduced as a plan for reform and investment because 'the NHS is a 1940's system operating in a 21st century world'.
  (The NHS Plan 'A Summary' Dept of Health July 2000 p 2)

Related developments include

- National Institute for Clinical Excellence (NICE) which aims to set standards in health services e.g. it 'will ensure that access to cost effective drugs like those for cancer are not dependent on where you live'
  (The NHS Plan 'A Summary' Dept of Health July 2000 page 4)

- Commission for Health Improvement (CHI), an independent inspectorate which monitors standards through inspection and recommends improvements
- Clinical governance, a statutory obligation under the 1999 Health Act for each provider to account for the quality of care they offer.

Clinical governance has particular implications for the individual nurse as it means accepting responsibility for the quality of care you give and improving care through evidence-based practice and your own professional development.

1.6.a

Find out more about the NHS and your NHS Trust.
Write your notes below.

You can look more closely at the organisation of your NHS Trust by
- **going to your hospital library**
- **contacting the Nursing Directorate**
- **contacting Human Resources**

Information about the NHS Trust is given out to all new employees and is usually discussed on your hospital induction programme.

1.7 The pluses and minuses of working in the UK

When you reflect on something you allow yourself a few minutes to put it into perspective and to plan how to improve things.

Think about

- How long have you been working in this hospital?
- How is it different from your previous workplace?

You can consider: your shift patterns, working relationships, procedures, documentation, support systems, your patients.

Some things at work you may be very proud of – new skills and new knowledge – these are the pluses.

Other things about your new workplace you may still feel uncomfortable about – these are the minuses.

1.7.a

On the table on page 31 – list the pluses and minuses of your new workplace.

1.7.b

Take one of the points which you listed under the minuses and think about how you could deal with it. Do you need more training in this area? Do you need to speak to someone and explain how you feel?

1.7.c

Take one of the points you listed under the pluses and reward yourself for achieving the goal of settling in to your new workplace or developing a new skill.

Today's date	How long I have been working in this hospital..................	
How is it different?	**+ (pluses)**	**- (minuses)**
Shift patterns	....	....
....	....	....
....	....	....
....	....	....
....	....	....
....	....	....
....	....	....
....	....	....
....	....	....
....	....	....
....	....	....
....	....	....

31

Unit 1   Assignment

Make a detailed plan of your clinical area

Step 1   Explain to your supervisor what you want to do and get permission if necessary.

Step 2   Draw a rough plan of your area and begin to mark the detail on it by looking closely and asking questions. Look at the Fire Exits and the location of fire equipment and ask any questions that might arise.

Make a note of any new abbreviations and acronyms that you come across as a result of your survey in My Personal Lexicon

Step 3   Ask to look in cupboards and locked rooms and note where things are located such as blank forms, brush and pan.

Step 4   Draw a neat copy of your plan using colour and labelling it clearly so that it would be useful to another new member of staff.

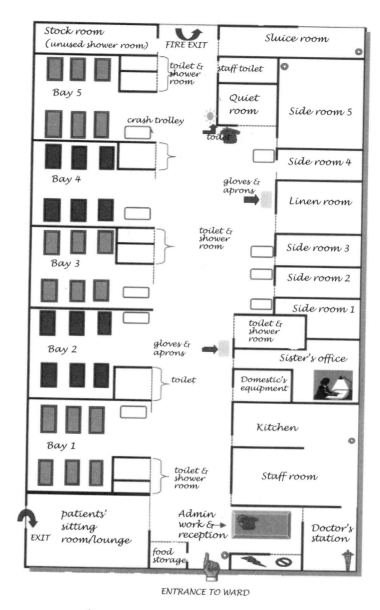

> Knowing where things are kept means you can find things for your team

Learning Objectives

On completion of this assignment you will be able to:

- locate equipment and fire exits

- locate where key people are to be found

- be more useful to our team

- ask questions (and answer them) more confidently.

2
unit

 Hello Goodbye
Words that stand out

 Taking phone calls

 Who do you know?

 Organisation of care

Make an organisation chart of all the
people who work in your clinical area

2.1 Hello Goodbye

How many people do you meet in the course of a single working day? Probably several
dozen. And with each of them, you probably have a slightly different relationship. This
relationship is reflected not just in the language you use when you talk to them but how
long you make each exchange. But perhaps the 'rules' for how much you talk to people
in the UK are different from your own culture.

2.1.a

**Think about daily life in your own culture. When you meet your next door
neighbour for the first time each day, do you:**

say nothing?

wave but say nothing?

say *Hello* only?

say *Hello* and some other comments, such as *How are you?* or
Cold today, isn't it?

have a conversation which lasts several minutes?

What do British people do in the same situation?
Of course it depends on the neighbour!

Here are ways of saying hello and goodbye in English.

Hello
Hi !
Good morning
Good afternoon
All right?
Good evening

Goodbye
Bye!   Byeeeeee!
I'm off now – bye.
Good night   Night
See you later
See you   Tuttie-bye
See you later, alligator

2.1.b

Listen to what your colleagues actually say at work.
Notice which expression is used in each relationship and write it in the
space under the relationships.

So the doctor might say to the nurse   *Morning, Sister*
and the sister answer   *Good Morning, Dr Jones*

Write down any new expressions you hear.

Nurse to nurse   Patient to doctor

Ward Manager to new nurse   Nurse to patient just admitted

Nurse to doctor   Nurse to patient who has been on the ward for a week

Doctor to nurse   Patient to nurse

Doctor to doctor   Nurse to patient's relatives

2.1.c

Write in the box below two or three experiences you have had at work in
the UK where the conversation stopped much sooner than you expected.
Who was speaking to whom? What was the exact relationship between the
talkers? Did the conversation stop for a reason (e.g. the phone rang)?

Where I was   **What happened**

Who was there

Stroking

Stroking is the art of saying just the right amount to a person in order to keep the relationship happy and functioning well.

Eric Berne in *Games People Play* says that the feeling you get of feeling happy and valued when someone says just the right thing is like someone stroking you. His actual words are *...stroking... denote(s) any act implying recognition of another's presence.* You can imagine a contented cat being stroked if you like! (Berne, Eric (1964) *Games People Play*, Penguin)

Let's go back to the neighbour situation. Imagine that you usually have a quick chat to your neighbour when you see them – maybe three or four turns like this:

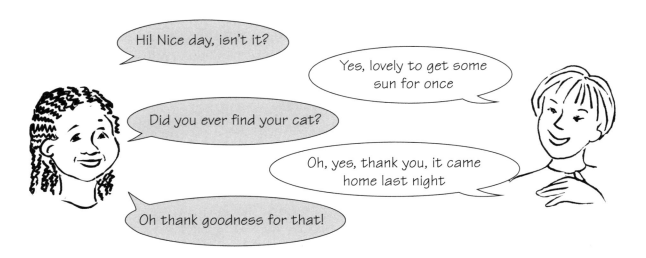

This is an example of stroking. It helps to build up the relationship.

If, instead, you just said Hello and went on your way, you might seem rude, or your neighbour might think you were offended in some way.

If, on the other hand, you suddenly start a long conversation with 20 turns or more, your neighbour will look at you very strangely! Why is she suddenly talking to me so much? Does she want something?

You may find that the number and length of turns that people in Britain (and especially in hospitals) use is much smaller than in your own culture.

Now look at your answers to 2.1.c. Do you think that knowing about stroking will help you judge how long a conversation should be to be comfortable? It may take a while to build up your cultural map of stroking.

2.2 Words that stand out

Look at the following sentence heard on a busy ward:

> ### We'll try and get him to theatre today

There are eight words in the sentence (nine if you count **we'll** as two!) but some of them are said more strongly (or stressed) than the others.

To say the word more strongly we can:

- make the word slightly louder
- take more time for the vowel sound
- lower or raise the pitch of the word

anything to make the word stand out from the others.

Try saying the sentence aloud. Which words are stressed in the sentence above? Why? You probably said the words **try, get, theatre** and **today**. Even here, **theatre** and **today** will probably be stressed more:

Why do we stress these words? Because they carry the new information and this is what we want the listener to pay attention to.

2.2.a

Which words would you stress in the following sentences?

1 *Have you spoken to the doctor?*

2 *It's in the cupboard.*

3 *It's in the cupboard on the right.*

4 *Would you like me to phone your wife?*

Sometimes the new information can change. There's a lot of difference between saying:

O

I've spoken to the doctor (stress on doctor) and

O

I've spoken to the doctor (stress on spoken)

Try saying the two sentences aloud. What is the difference in meaning between them?

In the first one, by stressing doctor, you are saying that it was the doctor you spoke to, not the nurse or the receptionist. In the second one, by stressing spoken, you are saying that you have spoken to the doctor, but you haven't seen him or her (maybe you spoke on the phone).

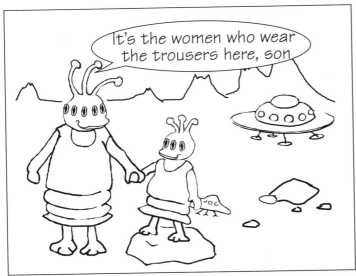

In the cartoon above which word or words would the father stress? Why?

2.2.b

Try saying the sentence below in different ways, each time stressing a different word. What do you mean in each case?

I'm not going to eat at Mc Dougals.

Match the meaning to the stress patterns below.

1 *I'm* not going to eat at Mc Dougals.

2 I'm *not* going to eat at Mc Dougals.

3 I'm not *going* to eat at Mc Dougals.

4 I'm not going to *eat* at Mc Dougals.

5 I'm not going to eat at *Mc Dougals.*

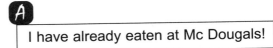
A I have already eaten at Mc Dougals!

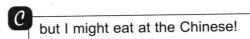
B but maybe somebody else will

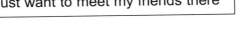
C but I might eat at the Chinese!

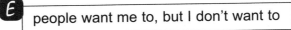
D I just want to meet my friends there

E people want me to, but I don't want to

When you record new phrases in My Personal Lexicon make sure you mark the stressed words as well. This will help you say them more clearly.

2.3   Taking phone calls

Do you find it difficult and stressful to use the phone?

Many nurses do – and not just international nurses! Some people hate using the phone even in their own language.

2.3.a

Read the passage and give at least three reasons why using the telephone is so difficult when you are speaking and listening in a second language.

Can you remember occasions from your work when communication broke down over the phone? Why did it happen? Telephone skills are difficult to master because you rely on listening to unfamiliar voices, reacting fast, asking the right questions and taking the right action. You cannot see the other person and it is hard or impossible to put an error right after the phone has been put down.

1   *There is no body language and you can't see the caller's face*

2   ....

3   ....

Phone Phobic?

Got a horror of using the phone professionally?

The easy way to start using the phone (again)

Follow these 5 easy steps and reward yourself each time you manage to complete a step. Take your time. You may be able to complete a step in one shift but, if it takes you a few shifts, that's fine.

Read this whole section through and then practise saying out loud the expressions needed for each step with your *Brilliant* buddy until they feel automatic to your tongue.

Don't panic.

To start with you do not need to **deal** with the call – simply to **answer** it!

Step 1 – bear with me

No-one likes a ringing phone. When the phone rings pick it up and say – without waiting for the other person to say anything -

Apricot Ward, Nurse Maisie speaking. Bear with me.
I'll just find someone who can help you.

Then go and find someone to deal with the caller.

Fill in your own details here:

Well done! You have answered the phone. This is the hardest part.
Give yourself a big reward.

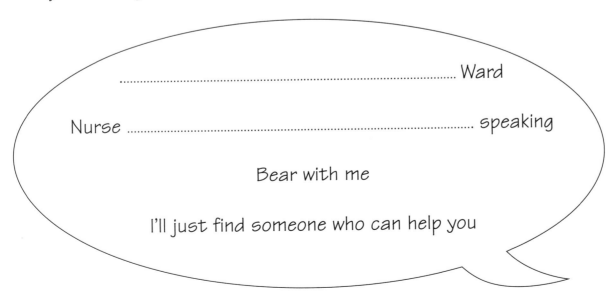

.... Ward

Nurse .... speaking

Bear with me

I'll just find someone who can help you

Step 2 – who

Find out **who** is calling and **who** they want to speak to?

When you have managed to answer the phone a few times using the *Bear with me* expression you can start to move on to finding out who is calling and who they want to speak to. Remember you are not trying to deal with the caller just to answer the call and help your team. Notice how you check the information each time.

> ....Ward,
> Nurse............................ speaking.
> Who is speaking, please?

> (It's) Mr Lowe

> So that's Mr Lowe speaking.
> Who do you want to speak to?

> (I want to speak
> to) Mrs Lowe

> So you want to speak to Mrs Lowe.
> Okay. Bear with me. I'll just find someone
> who can help you

Good work! You have identified the caller and passed the caller to someone who can help him or her.

Now remember to reward yourself.

Step 3 – taking a message

To build up your confidence you want to deal with an easy phone problem first. So when it is a question of taking a message for someone who is not there, try Step 3.

Read out loud the following call. See how you, the nurse, can take control of the call. You control the questions and the way the call develops.

.…….................Ward,
Nurse.…….......…...……..…. speaking.
Who is speaking, please?

(It's) Mr Lowe

So that's Mr Lowe speaking. Who do you want to speak to?

(I want to speak to) Mrs Lowe

So you want to speak to Mrs Lowe. I'm sorry she is not here at the moment. Can I take a message?

Yes – Tell her to ring me before 5

Can you spell her name for me?

L–O–W–E

What is your contact number?

0208 876 25432

Let me read that back to you
0208 876 25432
Is that okay?

Yes – Tell her to ring
me before 5

So you want Mrs Lowe to ring
you on this number before 5 o'clock?
I'll leave her the message

Thank you

You're welcome

Remember to check all the details with the caller at each stage. It is too late once the caller has put the phone down!

Complete the Message Pad below for the phone call in Step 3. Try this for real. Taking down a good accurate message can be a great help to your team.
Reward yourself for making a really big effort.

PHONE MESSAGE		
Date _June 30th_	Time _4.45 pm_	
From _____	To _____	
Delete as appropriate: Urgent/return call/for information only		
MESSAGE		
Message taken by _____		
Signed _____		

43

Step 4 – dealing with a routine call

Now you have some confidence in answering the phone.

Now you want to deal with the matter and give some information to another department. Let's assume you know the caller's voice and the call is a routine one.

...........................Ward,
Nurse................................. speaking.
Who is speaking, please?

Dr Henderson here

How can I help you Doctor?

Can you let me know how's Mrs Selby doing?

So you want to know how Mrs Selby is doing. Bear with me. I'll just go and look at her notes. She's tolerating fluids and has had some soup at lunch time. Her obs are stable

Okay. Bleep if there's any change

So you want us to bleep you if anything changes with Mrs Selby? I'll make a note on her record

Thanks

You're welcome

Remember the checking back is very important.
Using *So* to introduce the checking means the other caller listens to you and agrees with you. If you have made a mistake the caller can repeat his or her instructions. If you do not repeat the instructions the caller may be uncertain whether you understood what was wanted.

It may seem slow at first but in the long run checking information as you go along is quicker and less frustrating than making a mistake!

Step 5 – the caller from hell

Sometimes you may be faced with callers who are impossible to understand because of their own accent or how fast they speak.

You may have to deal with people who become rude when they hear a non-English accent.

Here are some ways of dealing with callers from hell.

Impatience

> Bear with me, please

Fast talking/difficult accent

> This line is bad, please speak more slowly

> I am writing it down, so please speak clearly

Rude

> I'm sorry. I don't think I can help you

> I'm sorry but I am going to get someone else to help you

> I think you need to speak to the Sister in charge/Ward Manager

You can always use the line you learnt in Step One.

> Bear with me. I'll just find someone who can help you

When you have used some of these phrases to handle a difficult caller you will be truly cured of your phone phobia.

Reward yourself and ask one of your colleagues to treat you to lunch to celebrate!

45

A word about your voice on the phone

Everyone's voice is distorted over the phone.

You need to use a slightly louder and stronger voice when you speak and also slow down your speaking by making the vowel sounds longer. This will make you sound clearer and more in control on the phone.

2.3.b

Try this with your *Brilliant* Buddy. Stand or sit back to back.

Try saying the directions below as if you were on the phone using the technique described.

a Breathe in, open your mouth slightly wider than usual and speak slightly more loudly.

b Make the vowel sounds longer to make the words longer which will take more time.

> This is All Saints hospital. To find us take the Number 8 Bus to St John's Square. Walk down St Swithins Street and turn left at the video shop. Carry straight on until you get to St Anne's School and our main entrance is opposite the school gates.
> St Barnabas Ward is on the second floor so go past reception and take the lift to the second floor. Turn right and you will find the ward entrance near the big bunch of flowers.

Think of this new voice as your 'telephone voice' and try it out. You may be surprised how confident this new voice makes you sound!
You might like to keep it as your professional voice for use in the hospital all the time.

2.3.c

You could write and practise saying the directions to your own hospital below.

2.4 Who do you know?

Although you may feel that you are by yourself when you first arrive, very quickly a new community of people is growing around you as you live and work in the UK.

2.4.a

Reflect on all the people that you know in the UK:

your patients

your social group

your kinship and family group

your community and church

your co-workers

How do they support you?

give advice, give praise, go out to eat together

2.4.b

How do you show that you value their support?

thank them, smile, throw a party

Discuss this with your *Brilliant* buddy.

If you haven't found a *Brilliant* buddy yet read page 167.

2.5 Organisation of care

How is the nursing care organised in your area?
Here are two models: Team Nursing and Primary Nursing.

Team Nursing

In team nursing a group of patients are assigned to a team which is headed by a Team Leader – usually a Grade F Nurse. This team leader leads a small group of qualified nurses, student nurses and healthcare assistants.

Primary Nursing

Primary Nursing is where a single nurse (often called the key or named nurse) plans and directs the care over a 24 hour period for a patient. In this care she/he is the patient's primary nurse. Other nurses on the team are then associate nurses for this patient. In his/her turn the nurse is the associate nurse for another patient.

The nurse's role includes admitting the patient, writing the care plan, evaluating the patient's progress, initiating treatment if necessary, working with other members of the multi-disciplinary team and arranging access to other resources.

There are other models of care organisation including **patient allocation** and modifications of these models. If you are working in areas such as theatres or outpatients you may be working with a particular surgeon or physician and their team. The organisation of care in these areas may be dependent on the particular skills and experience of the nurses and the types of cases or clinics dealt with.

How is care organised in your area?

2.5.a

Consider the pluses and minuses of the organisation of care in your area.

Where I work such as theatres, Ward 6

How care is organised here

What are the pluses and minuses for

the patient	the nurse	the organisation

Talk about this with your *Brilliant* buddy.

2.5.b

Which other nurses or health professionals are assigned to your area or visit on a regular basis?

Start to collect the names and titles of all the people who regularly work in or visit your area.

Introduce yourself and check their names and titles for your list.

Don't forget porters, cleaners, catering assistants and volunteers.

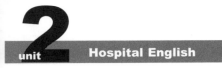
Unit 2 Assignment

Make an organisation chart of all the people who work in your clinical area

Step 1

Make a list of names and job titles.

Step 2

Create a chart with lines showing the organisational relationship between the staff members.

The chart should show visually how all the people relate to each other like a family tree. Are some staff line managers to others, such as ward managers? Are some staff who visit your area shared by the whole hospital — such as the infection control nurse?

Step 3

Make your chart as clear as possible.

Step 4

Check your chart is accurate with a senior staff member.

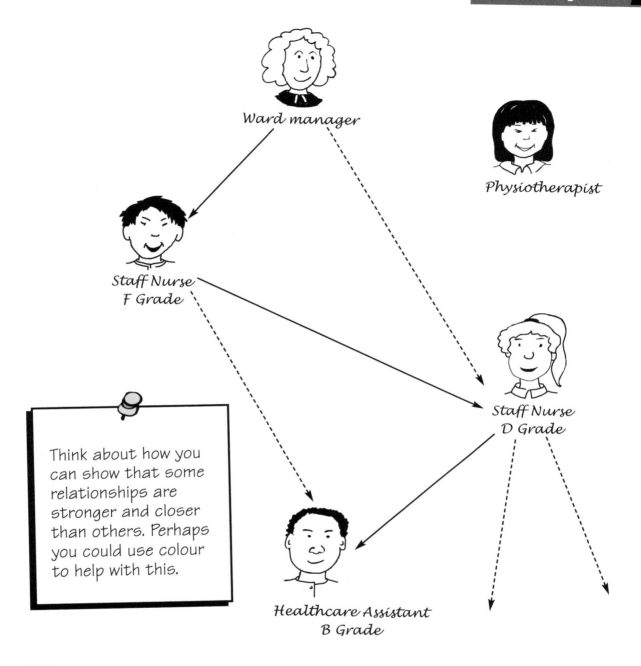

Ward manager

Physiotherapist

Staff Nurse
F Grade

Staff Nurse
D Grade

Think about how you
can show that some
relationships are
stronger and closer
than others. Perhaps
you could use colour
to help with this.

Healthcare Assistant
B Grade

Learning Objectives

After this assignment you will be able to:

- greet by name the people who work in your area

- understand the working relationships and roles in the area

- direct people confidently to the right person.

51

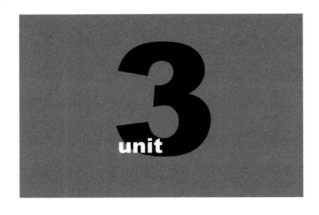

 Intonation's important, innit?
What use is a dictionary?
Sub-technical language

 Admitting your patient

 Maria's story - Asking your
supervisor for feedback

 Kolb and reflective learning

 Create a user guide for a piece of
equipment

3.1 Intonation's important, innit?

There are three intonation patterns which are common in English. You may already have begun to get familiar with them. These are easily heard in question forms and question tags:

The fall-rise

You're Lisa, aren't you?

This requires an answer because the intonation pattern shows you are not sure if this is Lisa. The answer would be *Yes, I am* or *No, I'm not.*

The rise-fall.

You're Lisa, aren't you?

This intonation pattern shows that you are pretty sure this is Lisa and you want confirmation only. The answer might be *That's right.*

The social snake

This is modulation up-and-down to indicate interest and encourage the speaker to continue. This intonation pattern is very popular in social contexts with any phrase.

Really.

Ask an English-speaking friend or colleague to say the three patterns for you.
If you can, record them onto a tape. Are you able to hear the differences?
Can you reproduce them yourself?

The most common pattern used by nurses in the workplace may be the rise-fall, or pattern two. This is used to confirm information from patients or to confirm a patient's cooperation in something you are doing. It adds to the sense of the nurse being in control and is reassuring.

3.2 What use is a dictionary?

Do you already use a dictionary? What sort is it?

Is it?

- A dictionary which translates your language into English.
- A pocket dictionary of everyday words.
- A fat dictionary full of words you've never heard spoken.
- A dictionary of nursing or medical words.

If you get the right one you have got a wonderful tool at your fingertips.

Another type of modern dictionary is one which is written for speakers of English as a second language and explains how people really use the language and gives examples taken from real life. Ask in your bookshop for the English as a Foreign Language (EFL) section where you will find these really useful dictionaries.

When you want to learn a new word or expression in a foreign language, what do you need to know about that word? Obviously you need to know what it means. But what else?

Usually, you would need to know

Basic stuff

1 (In writing) How to spell the word.
2 (In speaking) How to pronounce the word.
3 Is the word a noun, a verb, an adjective etc?

How is the word used?

4 Where did you first hear the word or phrase and who said it to whom?
5 Does it have any other uses or meanings?
6 Does it have special cultural meanings and associations?
7 Could it be offensive if used wrongly?

Not in the dictionary?

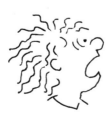

Not everything you hear in the hospital will be in the dictionary! There is a lot of modern spoken English which is so new that it hasn't had time to get into any dictionary!

WARNING

3.2.a

Here are eleven extracts from a learner's dictionary. The key information is in bold. Match the key information to the eleven categories below.

A good dictionary provides all this information or you could ask a colleague who knows it all.

A   rely **on** somebody/something

1   How to spell the word.

2   How to pronounce the word.

B   drip **n**

     pavement BrE the path you walk on at the side of the road **C**   **SIDEWALK AmE**

3   Whether the word is a noun, a verb, an adjective etc.

4   Whether the word is used in formal situations or informal, or both.

D

colour BrE, **color** AmE

5   The grammar of the word.

E   public school **BrE an expensive school** that parents pay to send their children to

6   Examples of the word in use.

7   Other words which commonly follow the word.

F   poorly BrE **informal** ill

8   If the word is an abbreviation or an acronym, what the full form is.

deal v **dealt, dealt, dealing**   **G**

9   If the word has negative or positive connotations.

H   pains /peɪnz/

     GCSE **General Certificate of Secondary Education**   **I**

10   If the word has cultural associations.

11   If the word is different in American, or Indian, or Australian varieties of English.

determined **He was determined to become an artist**   **J**

v	=	verb
n	=	noun
AmE	=	American English
BrE	=	British English

complacent (**usually disapproving**) too satisfied with yourself or with **K**   a situation

3.3 Sub-technical language

There are many words which are used in everyday life, but have a special meaning when they are used in the hospital.

For example, what can the word drip mean?

1 An unconfident foolish young man
(colloquial - negative) *He's a right 'drip'.*

2 A continuous dropping of water from a tap
(general) *That tap 'drips' all night.*

3 Equipment which instills a medication drop by drop
(nursing) *Have you checked the 'drip'?*

Drip is one example, but there are many others. We call this language sub-technical language: it is half-way between general usage and highly technical medical language. It is often the cause of communication breakdown between native and non-native speakers, or between users of American and British English, for example.

When you write words down in your lexicon, how can you distinguish between general and sub-technical uses of a word? What problems have you faced or can you predict in the use of sub-technical language in your work?

3.3.a

Complete the grid with general and sub-technical meanings for the words in the left-hand column. Then add some more from your own experience.

Word	General usage	Medical usage
Dressing	*Putting your clothes on*	*An antiseptic covering for a wound*
Stitches		
Sterile		
Addict		
Evacuation		
Collapse		
Pain		

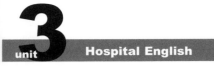
3.4   Admitting your patients

Most of you have to admit patients to your ward and there are many variations in the role of the nurse in admission.

You usually have to ask a lot of questions to complete an admission. A comprehensive and accurate assessment helps you formulate a good care plan and deliver appropriate and efficient nursing care.

If you work on a day surgery unit you will be spending a lot less time admitting a patient than if they are having major surgery. If a patient is chronically or critically ill and is likely to be an inpatient for some time you will spend considerably more time with that patient and perhaps their family. Admission can be an enjoyable task because you can get to know the patient, their history and to some extent their future expectations.

Some patients may have attended a pre-admission clinic and so will have given and received a great deal of information already. Some wards have a nurse specifically responsible for admissions who will handover a patient to the ward nurse. The admission procedure varies according to where you are working. There may be a General Admission form. In addition you may have a Manual Handling Assessment, a Nutritional Assessment and a Discharge Trigger form to name but a few.

3.4.a

List the names of any more forms that you have seen in your area

Asking for time

Do you have enough time to admit a patient? Work with your colleagues to share the workload so you can give your attention to the admission.

You may need to ask your colleagues for help in caring for your patients whilst you do an admission.

3.4.b

Write down three more phrases you can say to your fellow nurses? What do they say when they want to share the load?

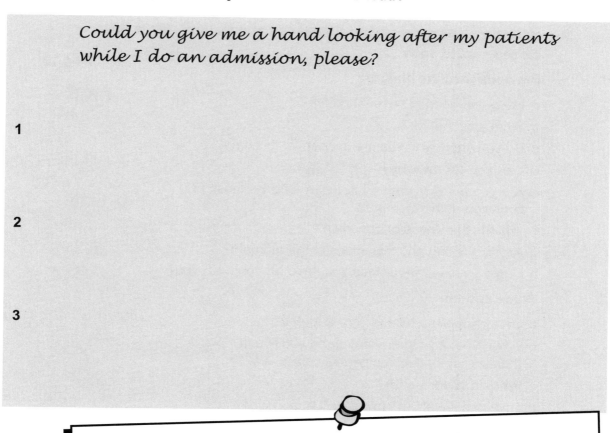

Could you give me a hand looking after my patients while I do an admission, please?

1

2

3

You may not be able complete the admission procedure in one session.

If a patient is tired and/or very ill you should ask a few questions at a time.

Many questions can be embarrassing so you should ensure privacy and confidentiality.

You may need to use and understand colloquial language when asking questions about sensitive subjects such as bowel habits.

Be ready to ask about any local words used for bowel habits and personal care.

Admission questions

Many international nurses find the most difficult part of admission is asking simple effective questions. Some of these questions should be open questions, others will be closed questions.

A closed question is typically a choice between two things, sometimes yes and no. There is no room for the patient to add more information. An open question allows space for the patient to add more information. Open questions typically start with 'what/when/how'. Questions on any topic can be open or closed.

3.4.c

Here are some examples of both types of questions. Write open or closed next to each

1   **Previous medical history**

    a Have you been in hospital before?   *Open*

    b What was that for?

    c Do you know why you are in hospital this time?

    d Can you tell me why?

    e Are you being treated by a doctor for any illness or condition at the moment?

    f What is the illness or condition?

    g Are you taking any medicines at the moment?

    h Could I see the medicines you have brought with you?

2   **Home and family**

    a Can you please tell me your address?

    b What type of accommodation do you live in? (house, flat, bedsit, residential home)

    c Who do you live with?

    d Do you have stairs in your accommodation?

    e Do you have family or friends locally?

    f Is your home near to shops and public transport?

3   **Eating and sleeping routines**

    a What do you usually have for breakfast/lunch/evening meal?

    b What foods do you prepare for yourself?

    c Do you have any special preferences or needs such as a low fat diet?

    d What food do you enjoy?

    e Do you usually sleep well at night?

    f Do you need any help getting ready for bed?

3.4.d

Give examples of both types of question in the table and add some more subjects to the list.

For the first subject an open question is best. However, your patient may have a poor memory, be disorientated or muddled so you may need both types of questions.

Subject	Open question	Closed question
Previous health	What illnesses or operations have you had in the past?	Have you had any illnesses or operations in the past?
Where they live		
Eating habits		
Sleeping habits		
Family		
Reason for current admission		

3.5　Asking your supervisor for feedback

THE SILENT SUPERVISOR

Maria worked alongside her supervisor everyday. Everyday they came to work and then went home at the end of the shift. Maria had a nagging feeling that her supervisor thought there was something unsatisfactory about her work. So one day at the end of their shift, she plucked up her courage, and found her supervisor in the tea room. 'How am I doing? I've been here three months and you haven't said anything.'

'Oh, don't worry,' said her supervisor. 'If I say nothing to you, that means everything's fine!'

Wherever you work, feedback is vital. You need to know what you are doing right as well as what you can improve.

'Until something goes wrong, supervisors often just keep quiet,' says Barbara Narakelia, a communication skills trainer. 'But positive feedback, praise, encouragement and simple information about what you're doing right is just as important as we grow into our new jobs. Think of it like feeding your confidence – no encouragement and your confidence grows very thin. So ask for feedback and watch your confidence fatten up!'

And that means you really have to go out and ask your supervisor for feedback.

But that's a difficult thing to do, especially in a frenetic modern workplace. It takes even more courage if you are working in a language and culture which is new to you.

'Few supervisors are trained in how to give useful feedback and they are always

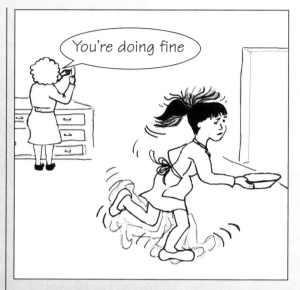

moving onto the next job on their list. ' says Agnes Magnet, a registered nurse. 'But feedback should be top of that list.'

'Of course', says Agnes, 'this doesn't guarantee that you get feedback. Your supervisor can always say 'Let's talk about it tomorrow' and never come back to you. But at least you have made the request, and it will be easier next time. She can't keep putting you off!'

After their talk about feedback, Maria's supervisor started to give Maria positive feedback at the end of each shift. She would say 'Well done, Maria.' This was very good for Maria's confidence but after a while Maria wanted to know how she could improve her performance and take on more responsibility. She wanted to know what exactly she could do better……

Why is positive feedback so vital?

Do you find you get more or less feedback on your work in the UK than in other countries where you have worked?

Here is one simple technique for getting feedback

The ABCD technique.

A stands for getting **Attention** You actually have to make sure your supervisor is ready to listen to you. Choose a sensible time and place. Make eye contact and use the person's name. Say something like *Peter, could you spare me a minute?*

If this is not the right time to have this talk wait for another time.

B stands for **Bridging**. It's important to build a bridge, a link, between you and the other person. This might be as simple as saying *Look, I can see you're really busy right now, but…* But don't spend too long on this – nothing is worse than a five minute apology for wasting a busy person's time!

C stands for **Communicate**. This is where you say what you want to say. It should be simple, direct, assertive without being aggressive, and as calmly factual as possible. *Could you give me some feedback as to how I'm doing so far?*

Always try to have a way to end the talk yourself – you can try thanking your supervisor for their time and saying goodbye.

D is **Development**. This is the way the talk resolves itself, perhaps by postponing until another time *Can we leave it until tomorrow? Say in the tea-break?* or by agreeing what to do next.

Can you think of two other phrases for getting someone's attention? Write them here:

....

....

....

In your culture, do you apologise for disturbing somebody?

How do you do this politely in the UK?

List some ways of ending the conversation

....

....

....

....

3.6 Kolb and reflective learning

You will find that reflective practice is quite a big part of nursing education and is considered valuable in the UK. Thoughout this programme we ask you to reflect on various aspects of your work and relationships and on your communication skills.

As you develop your new professional identity and take on more responsibility you will be changing. The National Health Service around you is always changing as new policies, procedures and equipment are brought in.

To manage change it is useful to adopt a simple system for thinking about it and making rational changes in your behaviour. This is the real environment of learning which is all around you.

This simple system is an adaptation of a model of the cognitive cycle of learning which was developed by Kolb.

The Learning Cycle

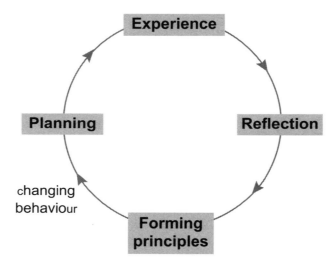

This cycle is in four phases.

Experience
This is where the activity takes place in real time – your experience of what you actually do.

Reflection
This is a where you observe the emotional responses you have to the event or activity which you are considering. It is a non-judgmental phase. All responses, good and bad, should be noted here. Be honest and inclusive. This phase you can think of as being from your heart.

Forming principles

Here you are beginning to rationalise your experience. This phase is where you have to use your head! You look at your experience and begin to evaluate your responses.

You draw lessons from your experience which fall into two areas:

1 what you must do to maximise the positive aspects of the experience, and

2 what you must do to minimise the negative aspects.

You are looking for general principles on which you will base your next actions. This is not a criticism of your past behaviour but a way of planning for the future so that you are more likely to be successful.

This phase is often easier if you have a sympathetic person, such as your buddy, to discuss it with, who can help you see the constructive way forward. You must not discount the negative reflections as they have a role to play in helping you plan better.

Planning action

This phase is the practical outcome of the thinking. Having worked out what principles you need to adopt you have to work out what action to take. Action-planning is simply new behaviour which you are choosing to adopt.

If you do not plan action you will find that you fall back into comfortable old patterns of behaviour. That is why there is the little note – changing behaviour – between these two phases.

So

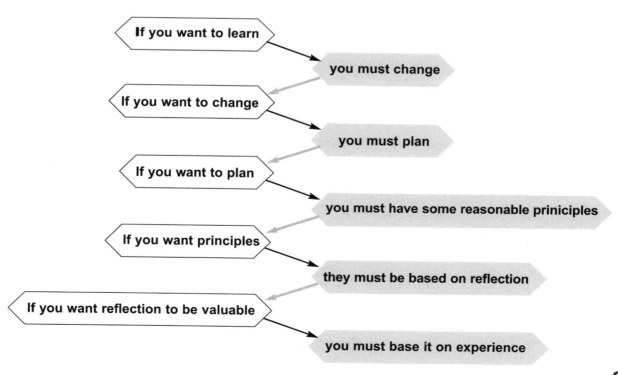

The learning cycle is one of the formats in which you can keep your notes.

Look at the example below

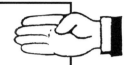

Buy a small bound book to record your reflections.

Call this My Professional Identity Notebook
– or PIN for short!

My Professional Identity Notebook

My experience

I am trying to learn about some equipment in my area. Usually I don't have time to write much. When I do write things down they are always on pieces of paper - I usually lose them and have to ask the same questions again.

My reflection on this experience

I feel - stupid having to ask again and again
- cross because I can't find the paper notes from last time
- not a useful team member as I cannot be left unsupervised
- okay when I remember to write things down
- okay because I have a sympathetic supervisor

What general principles can I draw from this?
(Changing my behaviour)

1 Writing things down in a note book will help me learn faster
2 Looking prepared when I come to use the equipment will help me feel less unprofessional

What am I going to do next?
(Plan practical steps)

1 Buy a small bound notebook for this purpose and keep it in my uniform
2 Get all my notes in one place and check them with my supervisor

Follow up

This time I was ready when we started with the new equipment. My supervisor helped me write a lot of notes and checked my understanding. I felt professionally competent, my supervisor praised me.

Sometimes you may feel confidence is given to us only through other people's approval. It is certainly true that we build our self-esteem very much on the opinion of others, but it is often possible by slight changes in our own behaviour to bring out more of this positive response in others. We influence people indirectly by how we present ourselves. If we present ourselves as competent and confident others may show their approval, which will make us feel more confident and competent. It is a virtuous circle!

3.6.a

Write notes in a learning cycle format for one experience this week which boosted your confidence. In your planning phase focus on what YOU can do to make more of this sort of thing happen.

My Professional Identity Notebook

My experience

My reflection on this experience

What general principles can I draw from this?
(Changing my behaviour)

What am I going to do next?
(Plan practical steps)

Follow up

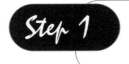

Unit 3   Assignment

Create a user guide for a piece of equipment used for moving and handling

Step 1 Locate all the equipment in your area which is used for moving and handling and choose a piece of equipment to evaluate

Negotiate with your mentor which piece of equipment would be useful to write a guide to.

Step 2 Draw it (or use an existing picture) and label it clearly.

Illustrate the equipment with

- drawings
- cut-outs from brochures
- photographs

Label the equipment appropriately, for example

- generic name
- common or colloquial name or nickname
- abbreviation if commonly used
- manufacturer's name

Step 3

Describe how it functions and how it should be used by the nurse and the patient.

Describe any training needed to use this equipment and where this can be found.

Step 4

Evaluate the design of the equipment.

Is it always used in the correct way?

Does the design have any disadvantages?

If you were introducing the equipment into your area what recommendations would you make?

Word count: 400-500

Sources of information

- Manufacturer notices
- Training materials and safety protocols
- Journals and books on moving and handling
- The back care facilitator
- Your mentor

You can laminate the illustrated guide and present it to your area

Learning Objectives

After completing this assignment you will know:

- what equipment is available for moving and handling in your area
- how to assess the usefulness of a piece of equipment
- how to explain to others how to use it
- if training is required, where to obtain it.

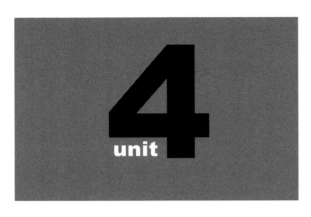

unit 4

 Short forms
Linking sounds together
Telling an anecdote

 Confidentiality

 How's your bridging?

 Acknowledging your limitations

 Make a profile of one patient's experience of hospital

4.1 Short forms

**LO RU OK
CU L8R
TTFN**

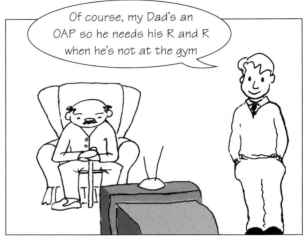

> Of course, my Dad's an OAP so he needs his R and R when he's not at the gym

Abbreviations are short forms of words, like Dr for Doctor. Acronyms are words made of the initials of a phrase, often the initials of the name of an organisation, so WHO is the acronym of the World Health Organization.

British people love to shorten words (as in the text message above) and it is useful to learn what the short forms mean. Be careful if you write down a short form in patient notes – it may not be understood. Some nurse trainers believe you should never use short forms professionally, for example in patient notes. Try to use full forms instead.

Record abbreviations and acronyms in My Personal Lexicon.

List them in a separate place at the end, or in a special section in the middle, so you can find them again easily

4.1.a

 What do the following short forms mean? If you don't know, find out! Write the answers in the box.

OT	=	
POP	=	
pt	=	
A&E	=	
RTA	=	
(r)	=	

4.2 Linking sounds together

Do you think it is important to speak in the same way that British people speak? Do you speak English with a strong accent? Does it matter? The most important thing is to be clear and intelligible.

One way of improving your pronunciation, and also helping you to understand British people when they speak, is to work on linking sounds together.

What is linking? If you say the two words *this* and *car* together – *this car* – the 's' sound from *this* moves over to the next word, as if it 'belongs' to *car*. This means you might hear – *the scar*.

If you then continue the sentence – *this car is* – you put in a new sound /r/ at the end of *car* making – *the scar riz*.

These sounds are difficult to hear in themselves, but can make the difference between understanding and not understanding, both for you and the people you speak to.

Here are three ways in which sounds are changed or left out where words meet:

1 **Change the sound at the end of the word.**

I've foun(d) the money

tem balloons (ten becomes tem)

3 **Add a sound between two vowels.**

You (w) are on the next shift

I (y) always wash my hands

Go (w) away

Africa (r) and Asia

2 **Move the sound to the start of the next word**

Get out – ge tout

4.2.a

Look at the following expressions and mark where there is a linking such as the ones described above.

a my mother and father

b DOA

c bed and breakfast

d road traffic accident

e have I ever told you about....?

f put it on a piece of paper

69

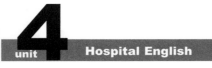

4.3 Telling an anecdote

Telling stories is part of every culture. Indeed, it is part of being a human being.

One way of passing on information about ourselves, or our relationships and the way things are in the world is to tell stories. Anecdotes are short stories which usually reveal something funny or strange about the way things are in the world.

Although story-telling is universal, there may be conventions about it which are different in the UK from your own culture: maybe some topics are taboo, for instance. And it's probably not a very good idea to tell a long anecdote just as the surgeon is about to operate – in any country!

Think of somebody you know really well who is a good teller of stories. What makes them so good?

> I'll tell you the most embarrassing experience …

I'll tell you the most embarrassing experience of my life. I had just taken up a job in England, and I spoke English pretty well, at least I thought I did, but of course when you actually have to speak to real people on the ward, it's quite another matter. Anyway, one day I met a new patient, I remember it was a lovely old lady called Mrs T and I asked her for some information about her illness – and I heard her say that she was suffering from donkey's ears! Now in all my medical career, all the books I'd read about medicine in English, I'd never heard of this, and naturally I thought it was some kind of slang, like athlete's foot or something, so I just smiled and then went to the nurse on duty and whispered 'Mrs T says she's got donkey's ears…' And the nurse said. 'I don't think so, my luv, I expect she said she's had it for donkey's years!' and burst out laughing. It means, apparently, for many years, or as many years as you can remember. How was I to know? I felt that small.

4.3.a

Listen to your colleagues telling stories and anecdotes at work and complete the following worksheet.

When do your colleagues tell stories and anecdotes?

- at the start of the shift?

- at the end of the shift?

- in the tea break?

- some other time?

What are the common topics of your colleagues' anecdotes? family? work? traffic? pets? weather?

Are anecdotes always funny?

Can they be sad stories or warnings?

Do they need a 'punchline' like in a joke?

How do British people

- **signal they are going to tell a story?**

- **finish their story?**

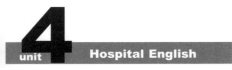

4.4   Confidentiality

Protecting private and personal information about your patient is one of the ways that a nurse can contribute to respecting and protecting patient autonomy.

> Clause 5 of the Code of Professional Conduct states.
>
> > As a registered nurse or midwife, you must protect confidential information.
>
> *NMC Code of Professional Conduct page 7*

4.4.a

Think about your own practice

Have you ever discussed the care you have provided for a patient outside your working environment?			
Never	once or twice	regularly	just to other nurses
Have you ever left patient notes open on the nurses station?			
Never	once or twice	regularly	no, but I know nurses who do
Have you ever left notebooks or sheets of paper around with patient details on?			
Never	once or twice	regularly	it happens now and again but nobody is really worried
Have you ever forgotten to provide adequate privacy when asking a patient private and personal questions?			
Never	once or twice	regularly	well, it isn't possible often to get privacy

You are not alone. It is likely that all nurses have done at least one of these things at some point in their professional career. However, if you have, you have breached confidence. Reflect on what happened and work out how you can prevent it happening again.

What is confidential information?

All information given about the patient from whatever source is confidential.

This includes personal and private details which might be given to you in conversation:

- even when you do not tell someone the name of the patient
- even when you speak in a different language
- even when you try to make written information anonymous
- even when you put patient notes away 'when you next have a minute' i.e. later on rather than at the time.

Who can you share information with and in what circumstances?

You can share information:

- with appropriate health or social work practitioners
- when it is used for the purpose for which the information was given
- with others outside the team if you have the patient's consent
- without the patient's consent if disclosure can be justified in the public interest, for example to protect the patient or someone else from the risk of significant harm.

In practice it may seem quite difficult to make a judgement as to what is necessary.

4.4.b

Choose Do or Don't as appropriate and then put a line through the wrong one. Check your answers with a senior staff member.

| Do | ~~Don't~~ | ensure that patients understand that some information may be available to other members of the team who are involved in their care |

| Do | Don't | consult with other members of the team if you are considering breaking confidentiality because you believe that this is in the patient's best interest |

| Do | Don't | talk about the care of an anonymous patient in the hospital dining room |

| Do | Don't | tell patients what is happening to the patient in the bed across from them |

| Do | Don't | ensure that, if patient records are taken off the ward, these are given only to a healthcare practitioner who needs them |

| Do | Don't | consult the patient regarding their wishes about sharing information with their family and significant others |

| Do | Don't | give out patient information on the phone to a relative or friend named in the notes |

| Do | Don't | give out patient information to a person who says they are a friend or relative |

| Do | Don't | check you know your own hospital's procedures and policies regarding confidentiality |

4.5 How's your bridging?

Interactional (I) communication and transactional (T) communication

You can talk to people in many different ways and for many different reasons but you can divide most of what you say into two main purposes for communication

transactional (T)	and	interactional (I)

Transactional communication: This is when you want to get something done: you may give an instruction or pass on some information.

This sort of language is not designed to build up relationships between people so people who mainly use transactional language may appear rude, bossy or simply unfriendly.

Interactional communication: This is language we use to establish and maintain relationships.

We like to speak to each other to see how we are all feeling. We greet people with language which is designed to gauge the atmosphere. We chat to show sympathy with someone, or to show an interest in them as a human being. We establish social groups and professional ties through language.

This communication is what you use when you are on the phone for hours to your loved ones. You may not have a lot of information to tell them but you do want to hear their voice and maintain the relationship for as long as possible.

International nurses are usually quite good at the **T- communication** because you know what to say to get your job done. But if you listen to British nurses you may hear a bigger mixture of **T- communication** and **I- communication**. Sometimes international nurses lack the confidence to build up their **I- communication** skills. But you need them!

You need the **I- communication** skills when:

- you are speaking to patients – so that your conversation is not simply a stream of instructions or information
- you are speaking to other members of staff socially in the staff room
- you are arriving at work
- you are leaving work
- you are getting to know a new member of staff.

There are many times when rushing in with your requirements may not get the desired result because you did not check whether the other person was ready and willing to help you. If you have not already done Unit 3.5 ABCD on page 61 try it now!

The B of the ABCD technique stands for **Bridging**. This is where your interactional skills come in.

4.5.a

You have to speak to a busy receptionist. Do you

a forget it and write the receptionist a note?

b say – *What's the phone number for Redbridge Hospital, please?*

c say – *Sorry to see you're so busy – this won't take a moment – can you help me find the number for Redbridge Hospital?*

If you chose

a good luck!

b **T- communication** – stating your problem but paying no attention to their problem

c mainly **I- communication** – recognising the receptionist's position, showing some empathy and stating your problem clearly.

The c solution is called **Bridging** – making an **I-communication** before jumping in with your **T-communication**.

In some circumstances you need to do a lot of **I-communication** before you can state what you want – especially if someone is having a bad day.

4.5.b

What about these situations? How could you bridge successfully here?

1 Miss T, 16 years old, is being admitted from casualty with abdominal pain. She arrives on a trolley. You are the only nurse available so need to work with the porters to move her onto the bed.

2 An auxiliary refuses to help you move a patient – she said she doesn't understand you.

3 A pharmacist gets very cross because you phone down to see if drugs for your ward are ready yet, and in fact they've been waiting for collection for some time.

There is no key for this exercise as there are many possible outcomes. Your communication should be successful if you have empathized with the other person's position, expressed your own needs clearly and negotiated a possible solution.

Discuss the situations with your mentor or *Brilliant* buddy and see how they would deal with them.

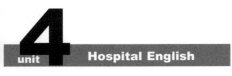

4.6 Acknowledging your limitations

Your 'scope of practice' means what tasks, activities and responsibilities you are allowed to perform within the law and professionally in the UK.

When you start work your scope is restricted because there are many new legal issues.

> The principles of Scope of Practice are clearly identified in the NMC document Code of Professional Conduct. For example 1.3 of this document states that
>
> You are personally accountable for your practice.
>
> *NMC Code of Professional Conduct page 3*

Being answerable for your own actions and omissions is a particularly complex issue for international nurses.

You are aiming to become recognised as a professional practitioner in a new environment, in a new country and to some extent working with a new language. Your scope of practice is likely to be limited for some time; we can look at some reasons for this.

The NMC's primary focus is to protect and support the health of the patient. In order for you to contribute towards this achievement you should be competent as defined by the NMC. Once you have registered you will continue your professional development through continual improvement of your knowledge and skills.

The Nursing and Midwifery Council's primary focus is to protect and support the health of the patient. Their motto is

> **Protecting the public through professional standards**

Some areas which were previously within your scope of practice may be outside it in the UK until you have done a particular training course. One example is intravenous drugs administration.

When you first became a nurse you began to make professional decisions and to use professional skills. These ways of behaving and attitudes form part of your professional identity. The attitudes include respect for and from your co-workers, trust, honesty, freedom to take independent action and to know and extend your scope of practice.

The next tasks are to help you reflect on your current scope of practice. Take your time, be honest with yourself and think deeply.

4.6.a

Identify five aspects of nursing practice that you previously fulfilled and that you are not permitted to perform in the UK due to your current status.

1

2

3

4

5

It is likely that you are being supported by a mentor or supervisor if you are in your adaptation or preceptorship period. You will be working towards the point when your mentor considers that you have demonstrated the required knowledge and skills for registration.

4.6.b

Identify three aspects of new knowledge and skills that you have recently acquired from your mentor or other staff members.

1

2

3

You cannot be good at everything and you may not yet have the opportunity to demonstrate your competence in all areas. Your workplace is likely to be very busy (as is your mentor). You may be aware of gaps in your knowledge and or weaknesses in your skills and possible reasons why you have them. For example, if you did not have to perform much hands-on personal care in your previous work then this may be an area where you are lacking in confidence.

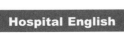

4.6.c

Identify three of your current limitations including those relating to communication skills or cultural differences. Next to each of your perceived limitations write one or more possible reasons for this.

limitation	reason
1	
2	
3	

You could use the list in Task 4.6.c as the basis of a discussion with your mentor at a future meeting. You should have many opportunities to take part in learning activities in your workplace.

4.6.d

Make a list of subjects that you would like to learn more about and say why – how would this make you a more effective nurse?

Look around your hospital for relevant information about Professional Development opportunities. Find out the telephone number of the Training Department, and the name of the person responsible for training.

4.7 Review

Well done ! You have completed half the units in this book.
Look back over your work and recognise that you are doing *Brilliantly*!
Reflect on any changes you have noticed in your communication skills and
confidence since starting the book.

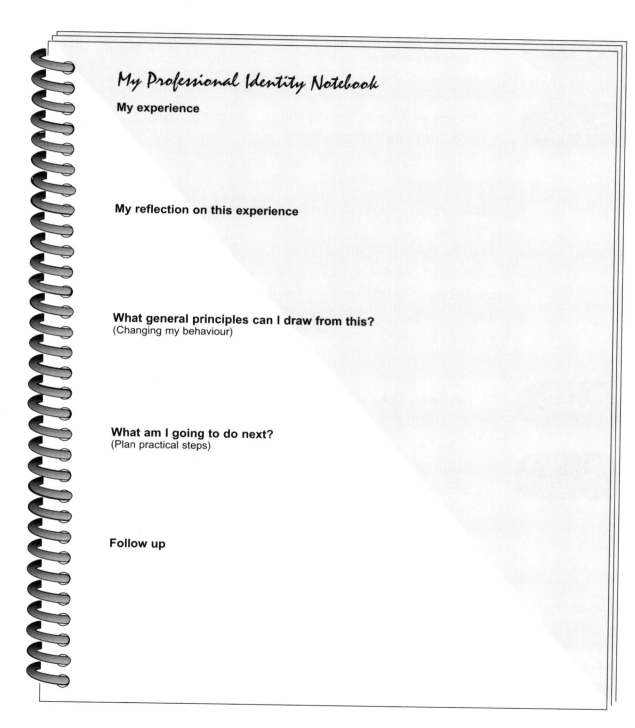

My Professional Identity Notebook

My experience

My reflection on this experience

What general principles can I draw from this?
(Changing my behaviour)

What am I going to do next?
(Plan practical steps)

Follow up

Unit 4   Assignment

Make a profile of one patient's experience of hospital

Step 1   Choose one patient who is currently on your ward.

Step 2   Check you are following the ground rules listed below.

Some ground rules:

- make sure the patient has given consent for both the profile and the interview
- get permission from your mentors
- explain clearly to the patient why you are making the profile and also, if appropriate, why you have chosen them
- remember to protect confidentiality. Make sure the record of all your data effectively disguises any individual identity.

Step 3   Interview your patient.

Step 4   Write up your interview in seven paragraphs.

1 A brief outline of the clinical details

Describe the patient's experience in hospital in relation to:

2 the treatment for their illness

3 being in the hospital

4 being cared for by the staff

5 Their expectations for the future after they get out of hospital.

6 Your evaluation of the findings

7 What you have learnt from the exercise

Format: you can choose the format for your profile. In any case, make sure it is clear, readable, and relevant. You can use headings, bullet points and so on, but do not write only in note form.

Length: up to 600 words

1. Brief outline of the clinical details

Mr Didot has recently had surgery for polyps on his gall bladder. He is 64 years old and has been reasonably fit and healthy in the past. He had a tonsillectomy as a child and has had hypertension for which he takes medication.

2. Treatment of the illness

'I was really surprised how simple it all was. Although I waited 7 months for the operation it went smoothly. I just have to visit the nurse at my GP surgery next week and come back for an appointment in a few weeks time'.

3. Being in the institution

'Although I hate hospitals I found it lovely, clean and not like I read it was in the paper.'

'It's actually quite nice to be able to chat to other patients, makes me realise how lucky I am.'

4. Being cared for by the staff

'Everyone was really nice. Sometimes I didn't know who was who, but then there are a lot of people working here.'

'The nurses were very thorough and I was surprised that they gave me medicines so that I didn't have any pain.'

5. Their expectations for the future after they get out of hospital

'Well, as I said i've got all my appointments sorted out, I hope that they go smoothly.'

'I'll take things easy for a couple of weeks.'

'The main thing is that I won't have to suffer from the pain that I had before the op.'

6. Your evaluation of the findings

It was nice to talk to a patient in more detail

It made me realise that patients have quite a few thoughts on their time in hospital

The patient had some negative ideas about hospital

The patient had a good opinion of the treatment he got on the ward

7. What you have learnt from the exercise

I've learnt that there are a number of rewards if we take time to talk to patients.

Learning Objectives

After this assignment you will be able to:

- feel confident in interviewing a native speaker

- have practised interactional communication

- be more aware to the psychosocial needs of patients in your area

- be better able to determine care based on whole-person needs.

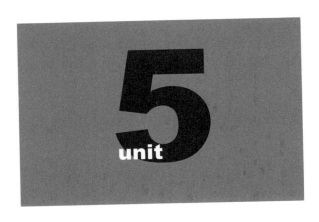

 Health promotion

 Handover

 Hospital diet lexicon
Making suggestions
Rhythm of English

 Interpreting graphs

 Prepare a short talk on a clinical subject

5.1 Health promotion

What does health promotion mean to you in your working life? It is important that we think of health and health promotion not just in biological or physical terms but also related to the psychological and social well-being of our patients.

> You must promote the interests of patients and clients. This includes helping individuals and groups gain access to health and social care, information and support relevant to their needs
>
> *NMC Code of Professional Conduct 2002 page 4*

There is much debate about what 'health education' is and what 'health promotion' is.

A leading textbook* identifies three strands of health education: 'Direct and individual patient-focused health education such as teaching a newly diagnosed person with diabetes about managing their diet and insulin regimen.' This is relevant to all registered nurses.

Another strand is 'consciousness raising' which we will also look at. The third strand 'targeting particular groups' is more directly relevant to nurses working in the community.

We are going to look at the first of the three strands of activity defined as 'Condition specific education with patients frequently focused on tertiary levels of prevention but also includes activities directed to primary and secondary prevention.'

Levels of prevention

Some nurses will be involved in giving secondary health education. This can be defined as action to diagnose early, to give appropriate care and treatment and reduce severity and duration of illness. You are also likely to be involved in giving tertiary health education. This centres on rehabilitation, recovery and prevention of recurrence or coping with a disability or chronic disease. In other words, tertiary health education is already part of our daily activities at work. However, as nurses we are usually

*Watson's Clinical Nursing and Related Sciences Mike Walsh, (Ed.) Balliere Tindall, (2002) page 16

dealing with the immediate needs of an acute illness you may need to reflect on how you can combine this with health promoting activities which often need some preparation and time.

Do you feel frustrated that you cannot devote adequate time to health promotion or education? Are you aware of the current approaches? Do you know what your hospital or area policy is regarding health promotion?

Your area may have relevant leaflets for patients and their relatives regarding care. You can use these as the basis of a discussion about health, recovery and prevention. When you give advice and information,

> You have a responsibility to deliver care based on current evidence, best practice and, where applicable, validated research when it is available.
>
> *NMC Code of Professional Conduct 2002 page 8*

Given that you may have a number of constraints it is necessary to develop strategies to enable you to carry out some health education activities. A competency framework may identify what knowledge and skills you should be aiming at. Find time to extend or demonstrate your ability in each area.

Health Promotion Competency Framework

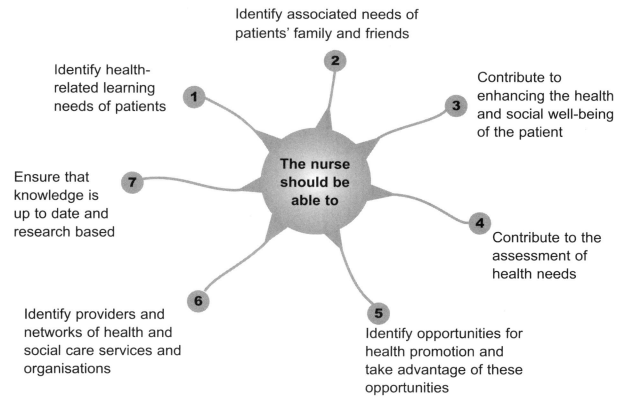

5.1.a

1   Write in your own words a definition of tertiary health education below

**2   Here are some examples of tertiary health education activities.
Tick which ones you have been involved in.**

☐   **a**   Encouraging patients to mobilise to the best of their ability to help prevent pressure sores

☐   **b**   Helping a patient make food choices that will fulfil their nutritional needs

☐   **c**   Encouraging patients to do breathing exercises or coughing as taught by the physiotherapist

☐   **d**   Encouraging compliance with medication

☐   **e**   Explaining an aspect of self-medication (e.g. a diabetic person administering insulin)

☐   **f**   Discussing possible reasons why your patient became ill (e.g. susceptibility to chest infection due to smoking or damp living conditions)

☐   **g**   Discussing lifestyle choices whilst you are carrying out patient care

3   Identify three tertiary health education activities that you regularly carry out in your area

a

b

c

5.1.b

Can you identify four difficulties or constraints facing a nurse in delivering health education?

a

b

c

d

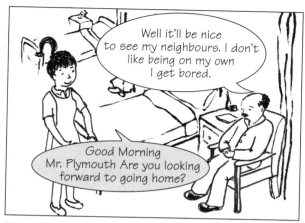

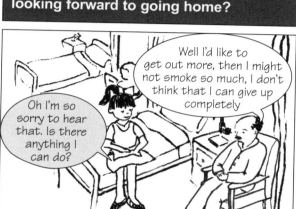

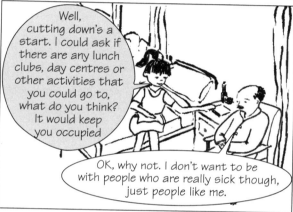

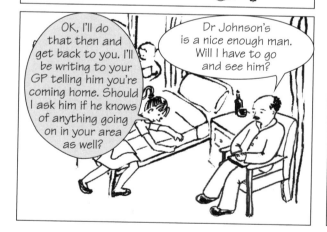

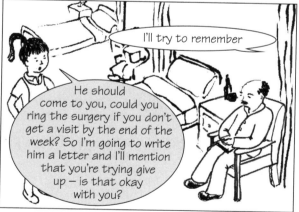

List any other materials available in your hospital that Maria might also give Mr Plymouth or his relatives to help him give up smoking.

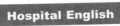

5.1.c

 A range of communication skills including cultural awareness and thinking skills are key to successful health promotions.

Identify which combination of skills or attitudes that you might need to be an effective health educator.

listening (L)	speaking (S)	writing (W)
reading (R)	cultural awareness (CA)	cognitive (thinking) skills (T)

1 Working with patients on an analysis of their needs and planning realistic, agreed targets

L. S. W. CA
....

2 Selecting information relevant to your patient and/or relatives

....

3 Translating or summarising health education information into patient-friendly language if necessary

....

4 Showing empathy (particularly if patient has not had success in changing habits or lifestyle)

....

5 Respecting your patient's beliefs or values

....

6 Being aware of learning models i.e. looking at different approaches as well as assessing your patients preferences

....

If you want to brush up these skills ask about any training and professional development around health promotion that are available in your hospital.

Make a note of who you should contact about professional development

5.2   Handover

You have now been working in a British hospital for a while. As you will know, one of the key events in your professional life is the "handover" at the start of your shift on the ward/unit. This is when the new shift is given a summary of the patient or patients and their care plans.

If you are working on a medical or surgical ward you may have a group handover where a senior nurse summarises for everyone what is happening on the ward and hands over all the patients.

Next there is usually an individual nurse to nurse handover, perhaps by the patient's bedside. Finally, you have some time to read the patient's charts, possibly listen and speak to your allocated patients, and check you have all the information you need before beginning your activities.

This section deals with building up your listening skills for getting the most out of the verbal handover.

The verbal handover is one of the occasions when you really need to listen intently.

5.2.a

What sort of communication problems are there during handover?
What are the reasons for these problems?

For example, when you first arrived in the UK, you found it difficult to understand native speakers talking at fast speed – or the nurse handing over spoke with an unfamiliar regional accent. Do you find it easy to catch numbers or details in the verbal handover?

What happens?

Why does it happen?

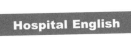

Listening for key words

It is very important that you try and get into the habit of listening for key words. In British English, the key words are said more strongly (or 'stressed') For example, in the following sentence, the important, or stressed, words are in capitals:

He's going to THEATRE TOMORROW MORNING.

More than one word can be a key word! If you are taking notes, it is simpler to write down only the key words not the whole sentence.

5.2.b

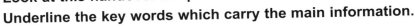

Look at this handover script.
Underline the key words which carry the main information.

> / second cubicle you have Vera Smith / she's a sixty year old under Mr Hartley / she came in with a trimalleolar fracture of the right ankle / she's for a check X-ray today / the form has been signed and taken to the department / she's completed her IV antibiotics / post op observations are stable / there's no neurovascular deficit / windows should be checked tomorrow the fifth of march and the back slabs to be replaced / she's going to be seen by the physio regarding mobility non-weight bearing / she lives in the bungalow with her family and she can go home when safe / and outpatients in two weeks / I have referred this lady to the OT for a general assessment

The number of key words is high because the person handing over wants to pack in as much information as possible in a short time. But you will find that these words are repeated again and again in subsequent handovers. If you notice them, write them down in My Personal Lexicon, and review them, you will be training your ear to hear these key words. Your ability to follow the handover should improve quickly.

5.2.c

This is a transcript of a nurse handing over in an orthopedic ward. Read the following script and predict what words have been left out.

Monday the fourth of March / Blue _team_ / first cubicle
Fred Bloggs a ninety (1) .... old / under Mr Southgate with
a (2) .... right neck of femur / alert and (3) ....
on admission / he has no past (4) .... history / he's
eating and drinking and (5)........................ / he's going to theatre
tomorrow morning (6)..................... he's nil by mouth from midnight

5.2.d

While you attend a verbal handover, take time to notice the typical pattern or routine in your area. Describe the order in which information is normally given.

Listening for patterns in handover

Here's another tip for improving your ability to follow verbal handover. Handovers often follow a set routine or pattern. In other words, the information about each patient is presented in the same order each time. As with telephone calls , if you can recognise the pattern, it becomes much easier for you to understand the information, because you know what's coming.

For example, if you know that the first item is always the location of the bed, and you hear 'first cubicle' you are more likely to get the information than if it is completely unexpected.

Here is an example handover pattern from the orthopedic ward.

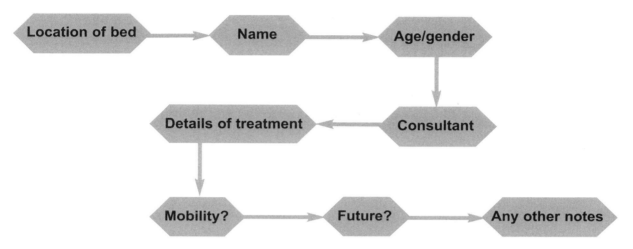

Use handover to write down the Key Words that occur on your ward.
You may need to stop the nurse handing over (politely! see below) to give you a chance to write the words and phrases down. Or you may want to find another nurse willing to identify difficult but frequently used Key Words so you can note them down.
Each time you do it, you will be familiar with more of them, so there will be fewer to write down. Listen and write. You can use My Professional Identity Notebook or My Personal Lexicon.

Strategies for checking and extending your information

Sometimes, you will not catch everything or some things you just won't understand. This is a fact of life: it happens to native speakers too. But it is advisable, especially in an important situation like handover, to have available some strategies, and some language, to help you. It is much better to say you do not understand, than to pretend you do, and make a mistake later. Also, unless you check the facts, sometimes you think you understand when in fact you don't!

Study the following expressions for checking and extending information. Do you think you could use these strategies at handover?

Typical situation

end of general verbal handover

Strategy

taking the senior nurse or other nurse aside and asking for missing information

> Excuse me sister, I didn't quite catch all of the update on Mrs Corn. I'm trying to listen well but sometimes miss things.

> Julie (your mentor) I'm sorry to say that I missed some of the report on Mrs Corn, could you help me out?

> Julie, I've read the report on Mrs Corn as I wasn't sure I heard everything. It said that she's doing well and that she should have her sutures removed today. Is there anything that I've missed?

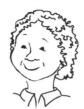

Typical situation

team discussion

Strategy

interrupting politely to check on the spot – note the use of name to get the attention of the speaker

> Paul, sorry to bother you I'm not sure who my third patient is, I've got Mrs Corn and Mr Costello

> Paul, did you hear the name of my third patient, I completely missed it?

> Paul, could you tell me which patients I've got, I got two of mine, but didn't get the name of the third

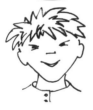

Typical situation

individual one to one handover

Strategy

giving feedback on the communication and asking for help for example - to a speaker with strong accent

> Would you be able to speak a little slower please I'm not used to a Scottish accent?

> You've got a great accent but I'm finding it a little hard to follow.

> Would you be able to repeat that last bit please I still have trouble hearing some things?

> I hope you don't mind me saying but I'm finding it a little difficult to understand some of what you're saying.

If some of these phrases seem useful to your situation, practise saying them out loud with the right stress and rhythm. Ask your buddy or mentor to listen to you saying them. Do you sound confident and in control? A bit loud and aggressive? Too quiet or passive? Now try them out in a real handover situations.

(Send the authors a postcard to let us know how you got on!)

Tense use in handover

Different cultures think of time in different ways. So different languages have developed different structures to describe the passing of time and when an action is finished or continuing, or whether something is now or in the future or past. Different varieties of English use the tense systems to decide action in time in ways which relate to their own cultural needs.

Analysing the use of tenses in handover, we can see common verb and tense forms. It is a good idea to notice the ones used by nurses on the ward and then use them yourself. This is NOT because British English is 'better' than your variety of English, but in order to save time, and also to help you be more comprehensible to your colleagues.

English tense use

Here is a simple way to spot which tense is being used.

1 Now

Present states and facts are usually expressed by the root form of the verb: *is/are/have/do/live*

She's sixty. Post op obs are stable.
She lives on her own. (fact)

2 Temporary conditions

are usually expressed by the continuous form: *is/are …ing*

He's eating and drinking well.
She's living on her own (at the moment)

3 Recent actions

especially where no specific time is given, or which are still true, or still going on, are usually expressed by the perfect form: *have* plus participle

Note   active form;   *has done*
                passive form: *has been done.*

The form has been signed.
She's got her TTs.

If the recent action has been continuous for some time, or has become a habit, we might add ---*ing*:

She's been vomiting throughout the night.

4 The story

of what the patient has done, or what has happened to the patient, including admission, is usually told in the past form: work= *worked talk =talked*

She came in on Monday.
He went for X-ray yesterday evening.

5 Future actions

are usually expressed by *going to* + verb, or *will* (usually shortened to *'ll*) + verb. Going to has more of an idea of something already arranged or decided (e.g. by the doctor). You also use going to to talk to a patient about what you are about to do.

I'm just going to give you a bit of a cough.
She's going to be seen by the physio.
You'll feel better soon.
We'll give him a CT-scan tomorrow.

5.2.e

In this exercise identify which of the five tenses is being used and why.

☐ **a** The doctor's <u>going to</u> come and have a chat to you this morning.

☐ **b** He <u>turned</u> his leg over when he was at work.

☐ **c** <u>I've spoken</u> to Mrs Avon's GP.

☐ **d** Sorry! <u>There's</u> no orange juice today.

☐ **e** <u>We've been waiting</u> to see the OT for over an hour!

☐ **f** <u>She's feeling</u> much better today.

☐ **g** <u>He's</u> no past history....

☐ **h** <u>We'll ask</u> John Carter to come and see him.

☐ **i** <u>There's been</u> no change during the night.

☐ **j** Yesterday evening the patient <u>reported</u> that his leg was aching.

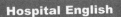
5.3 Hospital diet lexicon

5.3.a

The following dishes are all to be found in hospital menus in the UK.

1 Which ones are

.... main courses?

.... first courses?

.... sweets?

a Cauliflower & Aubergine Masala with Boiled Rice

b Orange Juice

d Cheese & Biscuits

c Bread & Butter Pudding with Custard

f Lamb, Bean and Tomato Hot-Pot

2 Which ones are

.... traditional British?

.... multi-cultural?

h W/Meal Egg & Tomato Sandwich

i Fruit Yoghurt

g Fresh Fruit

3 Which ones are suitable for

.... vegetarians?

.... diabetics?

j Minced Beef and Dumplings

e Saltfish & Calaloo with Rice

Food quiz

1 A traditional English breakfast includes the following items: eggs, bacon, toast, sausages, mushrooms, baked beans.
(true) false

2 Tea is usually served with sugar and lemon.
true   false

3 A British politician recently said that chicken tikka masala is now the national dish.
true   false

4 In Scotland, a 'takeaway' meal is often called a 'carry-out'.
true   false

5 Black pudding is not a sweet pudding at all, but a kind of sausage made from pig's blood.
true   false

6 British people are not allowed to drink coffee after 6pm
true   false

5.3.b

How much do you know about British food and drink? Answer True or False to the questions in the box.

5.3.c

Odd Man Out

Look at the four dishes in each box. Which one is the odd man out? The clue is in brackets.

1

macaroni cheese

ice cream

sunflower spread

rice pudding

(cows are involved)

2

braised beef with mushrooms

cabbage

hot sweet of the day

corned beef salad

(includes vegetables)

3

spicy chicken with rice

fresh fruit

vegetable soup

fruit yoghurt

(can be eaten by someone who can't chew)

Interacting with patients

Patients are very keen to talk to you about food! For this reason, and others, it is important for you to develop a store of useful language about food.

5.3.d

Here is some useful hospital English about food. Which phrases would be said by the patient to the nurse, and which by the nurse to the patient? Mark each one with P>N or N>P in the box.
Where the patient is speaking, how would you reply?

1   Would you like soup or fruit juice?

2   I'm a veggie

3   Shall I see if I can get you a specially made-up snack-box?*

4   What do you normally eat?

5   Do you have your main meal in the evening or at lunchtime?

6   It hurts me to swallow.

7   What do you think?

8   Can I bring in something for my husband?

* some hospitals will provide this service. Check if your hospital or ward does.

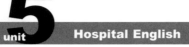
5.3.e

Here are seven typical questions patients might ask you about the menu but they may not use these grammatical correct phrases. Match the phrases below to the same question expressed in more colloquial English.

1 What's in it?

2 What does it taste like?

3 Is it a vegetarian dish?

4 Is it suitable for diabetics?

5 Is it very hot*?

6 Which one should I choose?

7 Am I allowed to eat X?

!

* NB hot in this context means 'spicy',
not the opposite of 'cold'

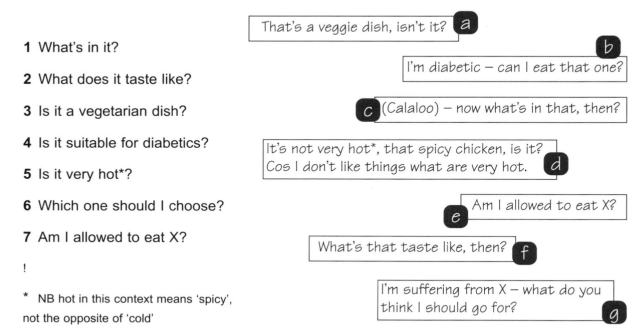

a That's a veggie dish, isn't it?

b I'm diabetic – can I eat that one?

c (Calaloo) – now what's in that, then?

d It's not very hot*, that spicy chicken, is it? Cos I don't like things what are very hot.

e Am I allowed to eat X?

f What's that taste like, then?

g I'm suffering from X – what do you think I should go for?

Apart from the question of what the food actually tastes like, you should know the answers to all the typical question for each item on the menu.

If you are working already in a British hospital, find a copy of your ward or hospital menu and make sure you can answer these questions about every dish! If you can't, who would be the best person to ask?

If you are not yet working in a hospital, try the same task using the two menus from British hospitals which are reproduced on p97.

5.3.f

Understanding hospital diet and patients' nutritional needs are a vital part of the nurse's 'knowledge bank'. What are the recent policy directives in your hospital regarding hospital food? What would you do to improve hospital food?

LUNCH MEAL

WARD NUMBER:

PATIENT NAME:

DATE:

Meal Type:

☐ **HALAL**
☐ **VEGETARIAN**
☐ KOSHER
☐ AFRO-CARIBBEAN

Menu Choices:

Starter

☐ 1 Natural Fruit Juice   DVS

Main Dish

☐ 2 Spicy Chicken with Rice   DHS
☐ 3 Curried Goat with Rice   DHS
☐ 4 Saltfish & Calaloo with Rice   HS
☐ 5 Lamb Stew with Rice   DH

Sweets

☐ 6 Fresh Fruit   DV
☐ 7 Fruit Yoghurt   DHSV
☐ 8 Hot Sweet of the Day   DS
☐ 9 Ice Cream   DHSV

MEAL CODES
H = High Protein
D = Diabetic
S = Soft
V = Vegetarian

These Dishes Contain Bones!
- Spicy Chicken with Rice
- Salt Fish & Cataloo with Rice

Name………………………..   Week 2
Ward……….   Bed No…………   Standard Menu Day 11
     Thursday Lunch

To order your meal please choose one item if required,
From each section and tick the box of your choice.

1	☐	Vegetable Soup	D♥
2	☐	Orange Juice	D♥V
3	☐	Minced Beef and Dumplings	D♥
4	☐	Lamb, Bean and Tomato Hot-Pot	D♥V
5	☐	Macaroni Cheese	DV
6	☐	Cauliflower & Aubergine Masala with Boiled Rice	D♀
7	☐	Red Thai Chicken Served On A Bed Of Rice	D♀
8	☐	Braised Beef with Mushrooms	D♥
9	☐	Corned Beef Salad	D♥
10	☐	White Chicken Roll Sandwich	DV
11	☐	W/Meal Egg & Tomato Sandwich	
12	☐	Creamed Potatoes	D♥V
13	☐	Boiled Potatoes	D♥V
14	☐	Mixed Vegetables	D♥V
15	☐	Cabbage	D♥V
16	☐	Bread & Butter Pudding with Custard	
17	☐	Rice Pudding	D♥V
18	☐	Fresh Fruit	D♥V
20	☐	Ice Cream	D♥V
21	☐	Light Fruit Yoghurt	D♥
22	☐	Cheese & Biscuits	D
23	☐	Sunflower Spread	D♥
24	☐	Low Fat Spread	D♥
25	☐	Butter	D

Portion Size   Small ☐   Large ☐

If you require sauce please tick box	
Tomato ☐	Tartare ☐
Salad Cream ☐	Brown ☐
Vinegar ☐	Mint ☐

MEAL CODES
*   contains gelatine
V   vegetarian
D   diabetic
♥   Healthy Eating
♀   NHS Signature Dishes

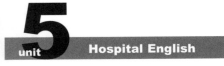

5.4 **Making suggestions**

You probably spend a lot of your time helping your patients by offering them choices of what to do to become more comfortable or to help the healing process. You have to be polite, persuasive and reassuring even when very busy.

Gaining a patients' cooperation is a matter of winning their trust by showing confidence in your own abilities. Clear instructions given gently can be reassuring. It is an important communication skill to be able to make suggestions to patients, and, sometimes, to persuade them gently into a course of action. Your tone of voice is important and so are your words.

Sometimes a patient is unwilling at first to do something that the nurse wants or needs them to do. Then you will need powers of persuasion – this involves gentle cajoling and good humour.

5.4.a

In the box are some ways of making suggestions. Listen to how the experienced nurses on your ward make suggestions and tick off any that you hear them use.
Write any other useful expressions you hear in the second half of the box.

If I were you, I'd …
eg, *If I were you, I'd talk to the doctor.*

Why don't you …?
eg, *Why don't you talk it over with your husband?*

Try + ----ing.
eg. *Try sleeping on your back.*

What/How about + ----ing?
eg. *What about moving it to the left?*

5.4.b

Can you think of two instances from last week when this has been the case for you? How did you deal with the situation?
Can you remember the words you used? Were you successful in gaining the patient's cooperation? Why? Why not?

Discuss what you have written with your *Brilliant* buddy.

Tone of voice

Some secrets of success

1 When you want to gain cooperation sometimes altering the tone of your voice can aid you.

- Lower the pitch of your voice
- Slow the pace down a little
- Use falling intonation at the end of the request
- Use 'please' at the end rather than the beginning of the request

This will help you stay calm, sound in control and matter-of-fact (not emotional).

2 Praising someone for making the effort to do what you want reinforces their desire to cooperate next time.

5.4.c

Listen to how your colleagues deal with patients who are unwilling to do something. Complete the box below for three different occasions.

What was the patient unwilling to do	Did the nurse manage persuade him/her?	How? What language did the nurse use?
get out of bed	Yes	Don't you want to have a little walk, Mrs Jones?
1		
2		
3		

5.5   **Rhythm of English**

Some people say that English is a musical language and should be pronounced with a kind of musical beat. This idea might help you with your own pronunciation. Stress patterns in a sentence can sometimes sound like music

I'm just going to see if he's answering the phone.

could be said with a beat like this: da DA da da DA da da DA da da DA

I'm JUST going to SEE if he's ANswering the PHONE.

Try saying it to yourself. Does that sound good?

5.5.a

When you learn new phrases, it is often useful to remember and even write down their rhythm. Look at the following idiomatic phrases and try and work out their rhythm. You can use the da DA da DA method as above or you can write large and small bubbles like this – o O o O

Can you match them to their pattern?

1	all over the place	**a**	o o O o o O o o
2	in the event	**b**	o O o o O
3	for all practical purposes	**c**	o o o O o o o
4	don't even think about it!	**d**	o o o O

Do you know what these idiomatic phrases mean and how they are used?
Ask your *Brilliant* buddy!

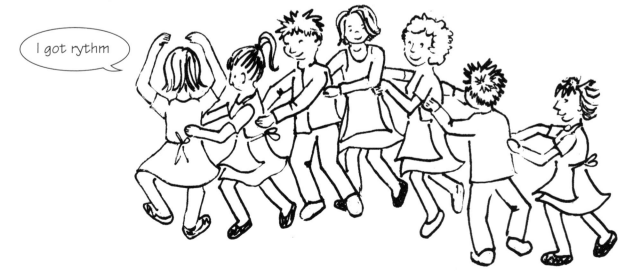

I got rythm

5.5.b

 Here are some phrases you might use professionally

1 to explain to a patient what you are doing

2 to get their consent for what you are about to do

3 to ask them questions.

How would you say them? Which words would you stress in these phrases?

1   *I'm just going to do your obs.*

2   *That's it!*

3   *Just pop yourself up on the bed.*

4   *Do you want to have a look at your X-ray?*

5   *Come and have a seat.*

6   *What we're going to do now....*

7   *Do you want to ring your wife?*

8   *We'll help you shift up the bed in just a minute.*

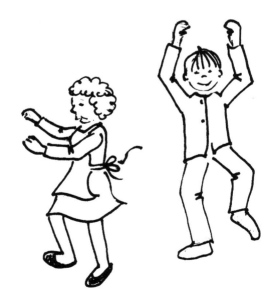

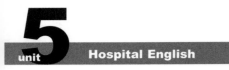

5.6 Interpreting graphs

Nurses often need to give graphical and statistical information in an oral report. These exercises are designed to help you interpret information quickly and use language accurately to describe what you see.

5.6.a

Look at the six figures on pages 103 and 104.

1 Which one is

a a table? ☐

b a bar chart? ☐

c a line graph? ☐

d a pie-chart? ☐

2 Study the figures for a few minutes to make sure you understand exactly what they mean. Can you pronounce all the

a clinical vocabulary

b numbers and dates?

3 What is the difference between **number** and **rate**?

For example, if a table shows that ten people out of a population of 40 suffer from a disease, then the **number** is 10, but the **rate** is one quarter, or 25 per cent (%)

Source of data for graphs and table:
Oxfordshire County Council, Health data supplement 2000/2001.

Fig 1 Proportions of minority ethnic groups in Oxford City PCT

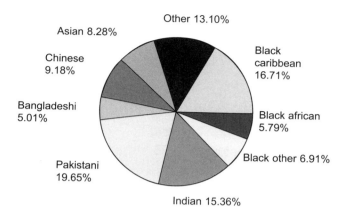

Other 13.10%

Asian 8.28%

Chinese 9.18%

Bangladeshi 5.01%

Pakistani 19.65%

Indian 15.36%

Black caribbean 16.71%

Black african 5.79%

Black other 6.91%

Fig 2 Total new cases of MRSA reported in Oxfordshire from 1996 to 2000

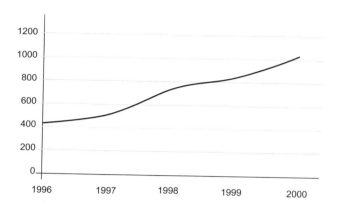

Fig 3 Cases of tuberculosis in Oxfordshire from 1974 to 2000

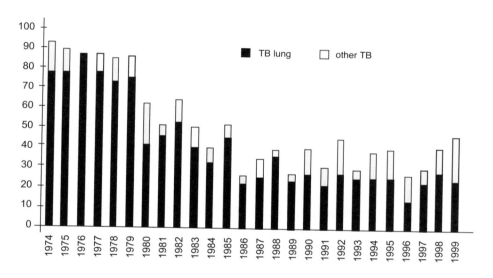

Fig 4 Cases of dysentry notified in 1999 and 2000

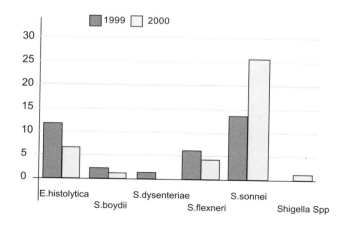

Fig 5 Confirmed or probable cases of meningococcal infection locally and nationally

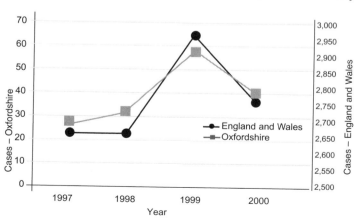

5.6.b

 All the sentences below are false. Correct them using figures 1– 6. The first has been done as an example.

1 The biggest ethnic minority group in Oxford City is <u>Indian</u>.

> *Pakistani*

2 There are nearly <u>three times</u> as many Chinese people in Oxford as Bangladeshi.

3 The <u>number</u> of dysentery notifications in Cherwell was 9 per 100,000.

4 The total <u>rate</u> of notifications in South Oxford was 335.

5 New cases of MRSA <u>dropped</u> between 1996 and 1997.

6 Cases of tuberculosis reached a peak in <u>1986</u>.

7 Cases of meningococcal infection <u>fell sharply</u> in both Oxfordshire and England and Wales between 1998 and 1999.

8 There were 11 cases of E.histolytica in 1999 compared with <u>15</u> in 2000.

9 There was a sharp <u>increase</u> in cases of tuberculocis between 1979 and 1980.

10 Oxford City had the highest number of notifications of notifiable diseases <u>but the lowest rate.</u>

Figure 6 Cases of notifications of notifiable diseases in Oxfordshire by district council in 2000

Number (per 100,000)	Cherwell	Oxford City	S. Oxford	Vale	W. Oxford	Oxfordshire
Food-borne infection	284 (199)	320 (228)	293 (229)	232 (205)	266 (267)	1395 (224)
Paratyphoid	2 (1)					2 (0)
Dysentery	13 (9)	11 (8)	11 (9)	2 (2)	2 (2)	39 (6)
Hepatitis	6 (5)	47 (34)		2 (2)	9 (9)	64 (10)
Meningococcal Disease	12 (8)	12 (9)	12 (9)	3 (3)	10 (10)	49 (8)
Other Meningitis	6 (4)	15 (11)	5 (4)	5 (4)	3 (3)	34 (5)
Scarlet Fever	1 (1)	4 (3)	4 (3)	8 (7)		17 (3)
Tuberculosis	8 (6)	28 (20)	4 (3)	5 (4)	1 (1)	46 (7)
Whooping Cough	2 (1)	1 (1)	2 (2)		1 (1)	6 (1)
Malaria		3 (2)	2 (2)	1 (1)		6 (1)
Measles		1 (1)				1 (0)
Mumps	1 (1)	1 (1)				2 (0)
Rubella		3 (2)	2 (2)			5 (1)
Giardia	21 (15)	37 (26)	26 (20)	13 (11)	8 (8)	105 (17)
Cryptosporidia	14 (10)	9 (6)	20 (16)	4 (4)	13 (13)	60 (10)
Total	**335 (235)**	**446 (318)**	**335 (262)**	**258 (228)**	**292 (293)**	**1666 (267)**

Useful language for describing tables and graphs

Verbs

rise
increase
fall
decline
decrease
reach a peak
level out
remain steady

Adjectives for describing increases and decreases:

slight
steady
sharp
steep
rapid
marked
significant

Nouns

increase
rise (in)
decrease
decline
fall
downward/upward trend

Adverbs

slightly
steadily
gradually
sharply
steeply
rapidly

Comparing words

compared with
...whereas....
if you take....
but..on the other hand
identical (to)...
twice/three times/100 times
as much/many....as...

Time expressions

in 1999
since 1995
for (nearly/just over/more than)
between 1230 and 1500 hours
during the period 1992 to 1997

5.6.c

1 The word 'increase' changes its word stress depending on whether it is a noun or a verb. Which is the verb? the noun?

   INcrease   inCREASE

   Practice saying these sentences with the correct word stress on increase.

   There was a noticeable increase in his temperature at 5pm.
   We must ask the doctor to increase the dosage

5.6.d

Put the words in the correct order to make grammatical sentences.

increase was sharp 1992 in there

1

a number has since the of 1990 notifications declined

2

relatively with 2000 1998 was compared quiet

3

Presenting information

5.6.e

Imagine you are going to summarise the information from ONE of these charts orally for your team. First make notes in the box about what you think is the key information.

Chart ....

What it describes

Main point 1

Main point 2

Main point 3

Something interesting you might like to draw the audience's attention to

Concluding point

Now you are going to structure a short talk or mini-presentation of less than 2 minutes.

One way of making a mini-presentation easy for your audience to follow is to have a basic structure or pattern in your mind. This one below is the most common on in English. To remember this structure you could write it down on a card.

1. Introduction - brief, state topic
2. Main points from the source information
How many? Depends on the info - not more than 3
3. One interesting point of detail
4. Conclusion
5. Check audience understanding

When you attend presentations and talks by other speakers, keep a list of useful phrases that the speaker uses to structure their talk. (Keep these separately from the content of the talk.)

Then you can signal this structure to your audience what you are going to say by using phrases like this:

1 Introduction

Good morning, ladies and gentlemen

Today I'd like to talk to you about…/ give you some information about…/ make a short presentation about…

As you know,….

This is a topic which has become…

2 Main information

The main point is that…

You can see from the handout/OHP/graph that…

As you can see from the handout/OHP/graph,

This is significant because….

A further/second important point is…

3 One interesting point of detail

One interesting point/detail/fact is + the…./the fact that…

You might be interested to note that….

4 Conclusion

To summarise …

That concludes my talk.

5 Checking understanding

If there are any questions, I'd be happy to try and answer them.

Thank you very much for your attention.

Obviously, the exact phrases you use will depend on the topic, your audience and the amount of time and information. However, the audience will recognise this structure and follow your talk, and you will be rewarded as an effective communicator!

Unit 5   Assignment

Prepare a short talk on a topic of professional interest to your team

Step 1 — Find a topic of interest to you in your professional life.

Remember you have a limited time to talk, only five minutes, so choose something which is limited in scope. One thing well researched and clearly presented is all that is needed.

Step 2 — Plan to give a talk to a group of your colleagues.

Decide how to present the main information. Use a visual aid if you wish. Do not simply copy graphs or tables! Summarise the main information from a graph - don't try to describe the whole thing.

Step 3 — Decide on a place and time to give your talk.

If you have a supportive ward manager, ask if you can present your talk at work – perhaps after a shift or during a staff meeting? If you prefer, make it more relaxed and present to friends away from work, for example at someone's house – and have a party afterwards.

Step 4 — Ask for feedback from your audience.

If you are working with your *Brilliant* Buddy you could take turns to give your talks and get feedback.

Research around the subject if you have time. You could use resources in your clinical area, medical library resources including electronic databases (your librarian will help you find the relevant sources of information) nursing textbooks and nursing journals, and discussion with nurses you come into contact with.

MY TOPIC IS -
handwashing

DATE/TIME FOR TALK-
Tues 4ᵗʰ Oct. 4.30-5

VENUE -
Seminar room, Ward 5

LIKELY AUDIENCE-
Ward manager, sister and anyone else free + my <u>Brilliant</u> buddy.

Learning Objectives

When you have completed this assignment:

- you will be able to speak to a small group with more confidence
- you will know how to conduct small scale research for clinical evidence on a topic
- you will have practised listening to and answering questions.

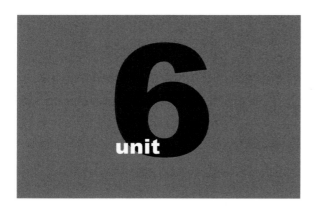

 Moving and handling

 Communication while moving a patient
Maria's story - Assertiveness

 Moving and handling lexicon
Word families

 Being part of a team
The ward round

 Interview two members of your team
Make a questionnaire

6.1　Moving and handling

Most international nurses are very surprised at the emphasis placed on safe moving and handling. All NHS employers have a 'safe handling' policy and most have a 'minimal handling' policy. The emphasis on patient and nurse safety has come about because of the number of injuries sustained when lifting and moving a patient, the amount of sick leave because of back pain, and in some cases the cost of legal cases. Advances in lifting and handling aids, safe techniques, comprehensive training and specific evidence based policies and procedures have brought about safer practice and happier nurses and patients.

The Manual Handling Operations Regulations (1992) states that the nurse should do no harm to the patient. It also requires employers to take steps to reduce the risk of injury to their staff. However, it is ultimately your responsibility to protect yourself from injury. This means that you should use whatever equipment is supplied and undertake any training that is available to you.

The emphasis in training is on:

- safe use of moving and handling aids
- protecting the patient and yourself from harm
- initial moving and handling assessment and regular re-assessment of the patient
- reporting any incidents.

When you start work, employers should offer comprehensive training from a moving and handling trainer. There should also be regular refresher courses. You may find named back care facilitators in your hospital. Their role is to disseminate information, give advice and promote good practice.

However, implementation of policies may be dependent on the necessary equipment being available and all members of the team putting into practice what they have been taught.

You may need to practise your assertiveness skills and be pro-active if other members of your team suggest using potentially hazardous techniques or are not keen to use appropriate equipment.

For international nurses there is the potential additional problem of effective communication with team members and with the patient. Assessment of the patient, information giving, gaining co-operation of both colleagues and patient and assessment of the outcomes of your action all require communication.

Listen to your colleagues and make a note of any effective phrases they use when carrying out moving and handling in My Personal Lexicon.

6.1.a

In your area locate all the equipment listed below:

☐ sliding sheet   ☐ electric bed

☐ handling belt   ☐ standing hoist

☐ bed ladder   ☐ banana board

☐ lateral transfer aid   ☐ wheelchair

6.1.b

Read out loud these phrases that you might use while moving and handling patients. Have you used these?
Learn and practise the ones you think would be most useful to you.

1   *I think that we should use the sliding sheet, OK?*

2   *Let's find out how much she can do for herself.*

3   *I'll just get the hoist.*

4   *I'd rather not do that, that's not what I was taught.*

5   *I helped her transfer on my own this morning but she's much more disorientated now.*

6   *What does it say on the moving and handling assessment form?*

7   *Have we tried letting her use the frame?*

8   *Let's get a second opinion, shall we?*

9   *What did the physio say on the ward round this morning?*

Finally some Moving and Handling Do's and Don'ts

DO

☺   assess the patient each time

☺   slide the patient (sliding sheets reduce a load by up to 75%)

☺   have a firm base

☺   report any injuries or near-miss incidents

☺   ensure that everyone (especially the patient) knows what is going to happen

☺   keep your knowledge and skills up to date

DON'T

☹   do the job if it's not necessary

☹   lift or drag a patient

☹   twist, stretch or bend

☹   continue to work if you have back pain

☹   use equipment if you have not had training

☹   try to move patients alone if the task needs more than one person

☹   be persuaded by colleagues to use techniques that you are not happy with

112

6.2 Communication while moving a patient

International nurses can find that doing and talking at the same time is difficult to manage. These exercises are designed to help you practise the language you need. If you can practise the situations with your *Brilliant* buddy you will develop greater confidence.

Communication strategies include:

decision making	*I think we should use the hoist, OK?*
gaining consent	*We'd like to move you with the sliding sheet, is that alright?*
reassurance	*I'll stay with you.*
persuasion	*It'll really help us if you can relax.*
encouragement	*You're doing well, great.*
movement	*Can you pop your leg up on the pillow?*
teamwork and co-ordination	*OK I'll say 'one two three, slide', are you ready?*
checking	*Is that alright now? Are you comfy?*

6.2.a

Make a list of typical moving and handling situations in your workplace
Put a star next to those that you find difficult (perhaps they are new to you)

Transferring a patient from bed to chair, or vice versa

6.2.b

Complete the table below with names of equipment you might use and an appropriate choice of language for each task.

Task	Equipment	Language
Helping a patient sit up in bed	*Bed Ladder Lifting pole (2 nurses)*	*Could you sit yourself up using the ladder then we can put your backrest into position?*
Helping a patient who is weight-bearing but frail move from bed to wheelchair		
Transferring a semi-conscious patient from floor to bed		
Transferring a drowsy patient from trolley to bed		
Transferring a non-weight-bearing patient from bed to chair (chair does not have removable arms)		

6.2.c

Take one of the typical examples of moving and handling that you are involved in and write a short dialogue which includes what you say to the patient and what you say to a colleague. Remember that you must also reassure and encourage the patient as well as giving instructions!

Share your dialogue with your *Brilliant* buddy and practise it out loud. You should be aiming for a good mix of **I** and **T** communication, clear instructions which are understood by your patient and colleague and a sense that you are in control of the situation.

6.2.d

What potential difficulties may stand in the way of using best practice?
List three.

1 ....

2 ....

3 ....

6.2.e

Using moving and handling guidelines or with the help of an experienced
nurse discuss some of the strategies you might use to overcome these
difficulties.

Difficulty	Action
Lack of patient co-operation	Spend a few minutes talking to the patient about the reasons for a particular procedure. Try to work out why the patient does not want to co-operate Try to plan ahead, offer your help to a colleague e.g. 'give me a shout if you need a hand and if I need a hand I'll call you'

6.3 Assertiveness

In Unit 3, we followed the adventures of Maria, an international nurse who was looking for ways of getting quality feedback from her supervisor. Here her story continues....

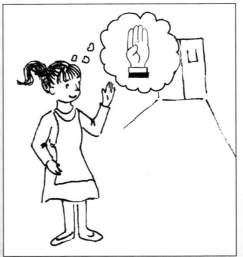

By now, Maria had been working on the ward for several months. She was a respected member of staff, though sometimes she got the feeling she was rather 'out of the loop', and that other nurses – especially the British ones – didn't give her the responsibility and respect she deserved. After all, she was the one with 20 years of nursing experience from around the world! She asked her buddy, an Indian nurse called Kusuman, for advice. 'You should be more assertive,' said Kusuman, 'I come from a culture where assertiveness is seen as challenging authority. But here you're seen as shy and passive. If you just agree with everybody all the time – well, people don't respect you. If you stick up yourself and explain what you need you'll get on better'.

| Do you ever get that feeling?

'Assertive behaviour can be defined as behaviour where you claim your rights. This does not mean being angry or aggressive: it means expressing yourself to others effectively.' So says Antonio Speranza, an assertiveness trainer from Harpenden. 'The weird thing is that if you bend over backwards to try and please other people, they end up trusting you less. Passive people (and actually a lot of aggressive people too) want to be liked by everyone – but you can't be liked by everybody all the time. The essential thing is to be fair.'

| What do you understand by passive and aggressive behaviour?

Two important rights in this respect are the right to have an opinion and to express it, and the right to have feelings and express them. In fact, just the day after Maria's conversation with Kusuman, a situation arose …

Maria and another nurse (we'll call her Elaine) were about to move an obese male patient, Mr T, from the bed to a chair. They were in a hurry, because the bed was needed urgently. Maria knew from the risk assessment that two nurses were not enough - the patient was going to be too heavy for them. One or both of them might easily damage their back. They might even drop the patient. Maria was thinking to herself 'we should be using the hoist – this isn't right'. Should she say something?

But Elaine was already walking down the corridor. 'Don't you think,' said Maria, 'we should use the hoist?' 'Don't be silly!' said Elaine in a joking tone. 'We'll soon get him moved.' With slight dismay, Maria saw Elaine disappearing down towards Mr T's bed.

| What would you have done?

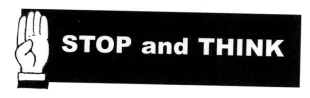

STOP and THINK

Maria felt she had three choices at this point.

1 The first thing that came into her mind was 'stuff this! Why should I be put in this impossible situation?' So she called out down the corridor 'I'm too busy at the moment. Can you get someone else?'

2 In the long run, she thought, the easiest thing to do is simply go along with Elaine. So she said nothing, followed the other nurse down the corridor, the two of them lifted Mr T onto the chair, and that was that. Next day....backache, of course, but which nurse does NOT have backache?

3 'I'll go and get the hoist,' she called out. 'There's one in Ward 6.' And off she went to get the hoist.

What did Maria do? And which of the three behaviours would be considered 'assertive' (as opposed to 'passive' or 'aggressive')? For the answers, look at the bottom of this page.

Maria went and got the hoist.

Speranza applauds Maria's actions. 'This is an excellent example of what I mean by assertiveness,' he says. 'Maria did what she felt was right; she didn't need to get angry with Elaine or put her down; she acted on her initiative, but in a cool, effective, professional way.'

Easier said than done! International nurses find assertiveness difficult at first, especially those who come from a culture where passivity is more respected or expected. But you will find that, in the British hospital setting, it is a vital part of effective working with others.

In Maria's story, there was a 'critical moment'. This was where the STOP AND THINK box was. This was the moment (as Maria realised afterwards) when she had to make a choice of how to behave, and try to behave in an assertive way.

In Maria's story the aggressive behaviour was calling down the corridor and refusing to help, and the passive behaviour was going along with the other nurse even though Maria could see it was a potentially dangerous course of action.

Below, you can see four useful strategies for taking action which might be seen as assertive when faced with a 'critical STOP and THINK moment'.
No. 1 was Maria's choice.

STOP and THINK

Critical moment – Strategy for appearing assertive

6.3.a

Write how each might help.

1 Go and do the job yourself.

It helps colleagues to see you as competent and doing what you think is right. This is sometimes called taking the initiative.

2 Change the way you are speaking.
Speak a little more loudly and more slowly, and make longer eye contact while you are speaking.

3 Change the place where the conversation is happening. Ask to move to a private office, or away from the bedside, or just down the corridor. Suggest this course of action.

4 Change the time that the conversation is happening. Ask to postpone a difficult conversation to another time or day if it seems to be going nowhere.

6.3.b

Think back to a recent occasion where you came to a 'critical moment'. It does not have to be one where conflict or tension was involved. This was a moment where you had a choice of which way to act.

Which action did you choose?

Describe the critical moment briefly.

Do you think now that it was assertive behaviour that you chose?

Or was it aggressive or passive?

What would the aggressive or passive or assertive choice of action have been in your case?

How do you now feel about your decision? Would you do it differently next time?

Read again the section on page 62 on the learning cycle which shows you how to use experience to improve your performance (and feel good about yourself).

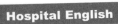
6.4   Moving and handling lexicon

Maria's Personal Lexicon has these examples of language relating to moving and handling.

Word/phrase/ abbreviation	Meaning	Examples/notes
1 history of falls	Patient who has fallen on previous occasions	Phrase used verbally or written in medical or nursing notes
2 PA's	Pressure areas or pressure sores	Commonly used abbreviation
3 risk assessment	Establishing potential vulnerability to pressure sores etc	Mrs Y has a risk assessment score of 7
4 I've done my back in / my leg's playing me up	Slang expressions for pain/lack of mobility usually due to an accident or injury	She's in a right state - she did her back in lifting a box - and now her shoulder's playing up as well
5 I can't get comfy	Can't get comfortable.	You don't look very comfy Mr Jones
6 shift up the bed	Move up towards the top of the bed	We'll help you shift up the bed in just a minute
7 Manual bed or King's fund bed	Most beds you will see will be this modern type of bed although there are now more electric beds	Also called high-low beds because they can change height
8 zimmer or zimmer frame	Metal four-legged frame used to create stability and increase mobility	I don't know what I'd do without my frame
9 O.T.	Occupational Therapist	Employed in hospitals and in the community
10 a bit wobbly	Feeling unsteady on your feet	I felt a bit wobbly when I first got out of bed.

6.4.a

Which of the phrases from Maria's lexicon could be used by patients (P), by nurses (N) or by both (P & N)? Write them in the box.

1 history of falls — **N**

2 PA's — ☐

3 risk assessment — ☐

4 I've done my back in
my leg's playing me up — ☐

5 I can't get comfy — ☐

6 shift up the bed — ☐

7 Manual bed or
King's fund bed — ☐

8 zimmer or zimmer frame — ☐

9 O.T. — ☐

10 a bit wobbly — ☐

6.4.b

Check you can clearly say the names of any special equipment you use. Mark the stressed syllables with a bubble. Write a sentence including the equipment to practise outloud.

1 sliding sheet

Have you seen the green sliding sheet?

2 handling belt

3 bed ladder

4 electric bed

5 banana board

6 wheelchair

7 standing hoist

8 sling

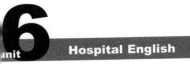
6.5 Word families

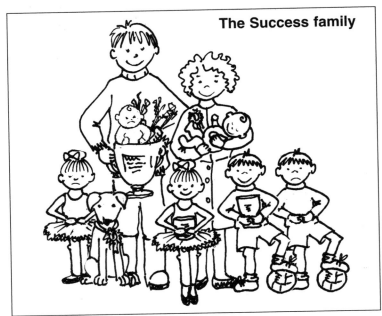

The Success family

When you learn a new word, it is very useful to find out other words which are in the same 'family' of words. For example, the word success is in the same family as these words:

unsuccessful

successfully

unsuccessfully

succeed.

When you note the new words down, make sure that you mark how they are pronounced. Sometimes the stressed syllable changes.

O o o
photograph

o O o o
photographer

o o O o
photographic

O o o o
radiograph

o o O o o
radiographer,

o o o O o
radiographic

This is of practical value if you know one word and need to use it in another part of speech, so you know the noun but now want to know the verb, if you are guessing the meaning of unfamiliar words, and in picking up everyday English which is often too new to have even got into the dictionary.

How do you find out these words? One way is to guess from words you already know by looking for patterns. For example, if the adjective *successful* makes the adverb *successfully*, then you might guess that the adjective *careless* will make the adverb *carelessly*.

6.5.a

Look at the examples, and then fill out the grid – look for patterns – they are easier to remember than individual lists.

adjective >> adverb		noun >> adjective		verb >> noun	
pattern ⟶ **add –ly**		pattern ⟶ **add –ful**		pattern ⟶ **add –ion** ⟶ **or –ment** ⟶ **or –ness**	
glad	*gladly*	care	*careful*	*reduce*	reduction
a peaceful	....	**b** fear	....	**c** happy	....
d	happily	**e**	beautiful	**f** encourage	....
g constant	....	**h** resent	....	**i**	equipment
j	ably	**k** hope	....	**l** action	....

I'm sorry to say that English is not entirely regular and these guesses don't always work. Sometimes the meaning of the word changes completely such as *hardly* which is not related to the adjective *hard,* and *life* which does not exist as *lifeful.*

Another way is to look in a good dictionary. In Unit 3 we looked at the different types of English dictionaries you can buy. We suggested you bought an English dictionary for speakers of English as a second language. These are usually a handy size and based on spoken as well as written English in use.

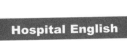
6.5.b

Use your English-English dictionary to complete the following table.
(A blacked out box indicates that there is no common word in that box.)

noun	adjective	verb	adverb
a	special	to specialise	specially
catheter		**b** to	
personality	personal	to personalise	**c**
d	social	to socialise	socially
imagination	imaginative	to imagine	**e**
f	active	to act	actively
explanation	**g**	to explain	explicitly
stress	stressful, or stressed	**h**	stressfully
gentleness	gentle	to be gentle with	**i**
improvement	**j**	to improve	
k	documentary	to document	
l	responsible	to be responsible to act responsibly	responsibly
accountability	**m**	to account for	accountably
n	infected	to infect	

6.5.c

Use one word from the table in the gaps in the sentences.

1 Washing hands is an effective .... control

2 My .... is in renal nursing.

3 If you want to .... your communication skills, practise every day!

4 Which person on the team is .... for the new staff?

5 Do you .... with your colleagues out of work?

6 He was skilled in personal care and was very .... with his patients.

7 Has the patient's treatment been fully .... to him?

8 He's a very pleasant man, but his .... hygiene is terrible!

9 He was laid up for three months, which was awful for such an .... man.

10 Remember to .... all your actions, including phone calls and relevant conversations with patients' relative.

In My Personal Lexicon you can leave space after noting a new word or phrase for adding the related family members in a quiet moment.

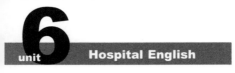

6.6 Being part of a team

When you arrive in your new place of work you will probably not see yourself as part of the team at work because becoming part of a team takes time. In addition, because you are new, your colleagues may be unsure where you fit in. If you still in an adaptation programme, this is a transitional phase gradually moving through your competencies or adapting your knowledge, skills and confidence. Remember that you are also adapting to a new culture and new communication tools.

It will help if you can reflect on your past roles at work.

If you find it difficult to assess your own role, talk through this task with your mentor. They can identify some of your qualities and how you fit in.

6.6.a

1 **What role did you play in your team in your past working environment?**

Ward manager ☐   Level one/newly qualified nurse ☐

Team leader ☐   Specialist nurse ☐

2 **What strengths did you bring to that team?**
Tick all that apply and add any new ones

Good listener ☐

Lots of energy ☐

Well organised ☐

Reliable ☐

Easy going ☐

Comprehensive knowledge ☐

My opinions are valued ☐

3 **What do you think of your current role**
Tick all that apply and add any new ones

I don't have much to contribute at the moment ☐

I sometimes say the wrong thing ☐

No one asks my opinion ☐

I am learning from some good role models at work ☐

I'm not sure what I should be doing ☐

I think it will take a long time to get back to the same level in the team as I was before ☐

I have got a lot to learn before I feel like a useful team member ☐

I'm worried about what people think of me ☐

4 **Are you using your skills and qualities to contribute to groups outside your workplace**

- Church or community group ☐
- In your house/flat ☐
- With your family ☐
- Social organiser ☐
- Your peers e.g. other international nurses ☐

5 **Who do you know in the team so far?**

Think about which people you get on well with at work. They may be people who are not in your immediate team e.g. professional development nurse, members of theatre staff, pharmacist.

List their names in your professional identity notebook and give reasons why you get on with them. Here are some examples:

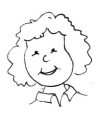 *Julie*
- Stoma care nurse, she's so approachable

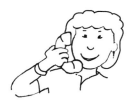 *Anna*
- professional development nurse, she's always there on the end of the phone

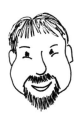 *Dan*
- pharmacist, he's so thorough

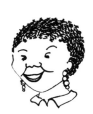 *Lily*
- shop assistant, she has a smile for everyone

The Unit 6 assignment is to help you get to know other members of the team.

6.7   The ward round

You may hear the 'ward round' called the 'doctors' round' but it might be more appropriately named the 'team round'. The ward round is one area where teamwork is essential. The use of the term 'doctors' round' is because it is scheduled around the most senior doctor's availability. It is a time when patients are reviewed by as many as possible of the professionals involved in the care and treatment of the patient.

The team usually arrive on the ward mid to late morning. The size of the team soon swells as nurses such as the named nurse and ward co-ordinator and other team members join the group. You might hear the phrase 'He or she is under Doctor Foster's team' indicating that Dr Foster is the consultant to whom the patient is allocated. A less senior doctor may take charge of the round if the consultant is absent.

If you are working in an intensive care unit you are likely to have a much closer relationship with others in the team as assessment and review will be on an ongoing basis.

From your experience so far use these exercises to reflect on your contribution to the ward round.

6.7.a

How free do nurses feel to speak to the team?

6.7.b

 What sort of contributions do the nurses make? Write down some phrases you have heard or would use.

6.7.c

How often do you contribute to these discussions?

6.7.d

If you don't contribute, tick the reasons that apply to you and discuss these with your *Brilliant* Buddy.

1   I'm not sure of the patient's condition and/or progress ☐

2   I'm lacking in confidence ☐

3   I feel my communication skills aren't adequate ☐

4   I'm new and don't have full responsibility for the patient ☐

5   I'm not used to working with such a large team – I feel overwhelmed ☐

6   I don't know who is who ☐

7   There doesn't seem to be an opportunity (fast pace) ☐

6.7.e

Give examples of the questions that nurses ask on a ward round.

Remember your rising intonation pattern should immediately alert the team to the fact that you are *asking a question*

6.7.f

In what ways is the patient involved in the case discussion?

6.7.g

List below some phrases you might hear spoken by

1 The House Officer or Registrar

2 The Physiotherapist

3 The Consultant

4 The Patient

6.7.h

The Ward Round has ended. What is your role now?

Do you need to ask the house officer to change the medication chart? eg There may be a white board for you to write requests on.

Do you have paperwork to look at, writing to do? eg You may want to check what has been written in the notes.

Do you have phone calls to make ? eg to the pharmacy.

Don't forget that there will be other times when you will be in contact with the rest of your team. Multidisciplinary team meetings are often held at least once a week and this is a chance to build relationships and learn about the roles of others. Eventually you may be invited to attend a patient review or case conference if the patient requires more complex input.

6.7.i

Following a round or team meeting write about your role and how you think your role in the team will change as you gain in skills, experience and confidence.

Is there anything you would like to change about the 'Ward Round'? Is it the best way of reviewing the patient's progress?

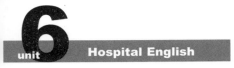

Unit 6 Assignment

Interview two members of your team about their pathway into the NHS

This assignment is designed to get you talking to other members of the team. You should find out how they got to be where they are, what qualifications they needed and what the pathway into the NHS was. You might want to ask how they feel about their role in the team and what qualities they bring to the role. You may find out some other interesting things too!

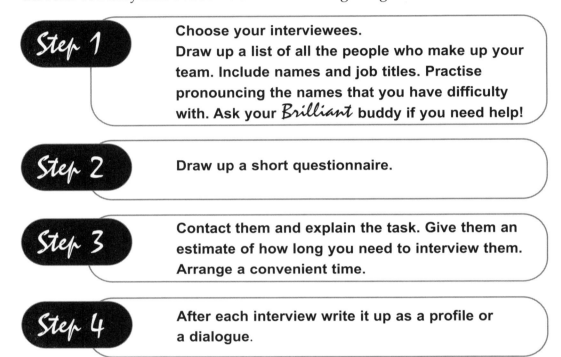

Step 1 — Choose your interviewees.
Draw up a list of all the people who make up your team. Include names and job titles. Practise pronouncing the names that you have difficulty with. Ask your *Brilliant* buddy if you need help!

Step 2 — Draw up a short questionnaire.

Step 3 — Contact them and explain the task. Give them an estimate of how long you need to interview them. Arrange a convenient time.

Step 4 — After each interview write it up as a profile or a dialogue.

We propose that you conduct a structured interview. To do this you need to design a questionnaire.

Making a questionnaire

Draw up questions for a short interview. You should ask questions about training and qualifications, special skills, and personal qualities necessary for the job.

Think carefully about when to use open and closed questions. Closed questions are useful for short answers and open questions allow the respondent to answer in their own way and at their own length. If you have time, type the questions out on a word processor and leave enough space for filling in the answers.

Before you start, try the questionnaire out on a willing victim, such as your *Brilliant* buddy. Then, if any questions are unclear, you can re-write them before commencing the interviews.

Now that you are satisfied with your questionnaire, use it!

ASSIGNMENT 6 INTERVIEW !

Nurse	Hello, Good afternoon, I'm Maria Thankyou for agreeing to talk to me
Clerk	Yes, no problem. I'm free now if you like.
Nurse	What were you doing before you came to work here?
Clerk	I was working in the waiting list office here
Nurse	What are your duties and responsibilities here?
Clerk	Preparation of notes for patients coming into the ward Telephone message handling Taking lab results Discharge filing and disposal of notes Entering information onto the computer system Arranging pre-assessment clinic dates and out-patient dates
Nurse	Do you need any special training and skills for this post?
Clerk	Nothing specific. my clerical experience in my previous hospital job helped me.
Nurse	Great. What do you like about this job?
Clerk	The hours are convenient for me. That is from 7.45-2.45p.m.. I get more time to do other things
Nurse	Is there anything you don't like about the job?
Clerk	I don't like having to tidy up when people leave notes and forms all over the place

Think about how, when and where you will conduct the interviews. It is probably a good idea to pre-arrange the interview, or perhaps do the questions in more than one session if people are busy!

Learning Objectives

After completing this assignment you will be able to:

- identify members of the team

- recognise the professional pathways of a number of team members

- construct a questionnaire

- conduct a structured interview.

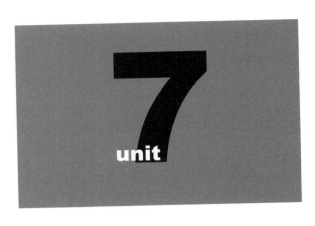
unit 7

 Transferring your patient

 Making phone calls

 Record keeping

 The legal framework

 Transfer of care in your hospital

7.1 Transferring your patient

Those of you working on medical or surgical wards will need to learn the complex and often time-consuming task of transferring or discharging your patients. This is an area of nursing that requires many different skills and quite specific knowledge of 'the way we do things here'. As time passes you will build up experience of forward planning, knowledge of local services and knowledge of your patients' needs. The exercises in this section are designed to help you focus on this information-gathering phase.

Right from the moment that a patient is admitted, the nurse and other members of the ward team are gathering information that may be needed when it comes to the patient going home. This is particularly important if the person lives alone or may be less able to cope independently when they get home.

Resource limitations may not be obvious until you try to access a particular service. You may reasonably make your recommendations based on your knowledge of the patients' needs but these decisions are normally taken by a senior member of your team. Patients' needs may be extremely complex – you cannot be expected to learn everything overnight!

Some of your hospitals may have specialist nurses in post who are experts in this field, they are usually called Discharge Co-ordinator or Discharge Specialist. They liaise closely with the relevant wards and should be able to offer support and advice. Some of you may also have a department called Single Point of Access (SPA). Here a single telephone referral from you will be the stimulus for appropriate action related to your patient's needs.

7.1.a

Familiarise yourself with the organisation of care for the patient in your community.

Find out:

1 what services are appropriate for particular patients in your area

2 what services are available in your local health authority area

3 how to access the services

4 whether there are any resource (cost) implications of accessing certain services.

Your job is to give as full a picture as possible of the patient including:

- their past medical history
- their treatment and care in hospital
- their current physical, mental and emotional state
- where they live and with whom
- what type of accommodation the patient has
- what other agencies and services have previously been involved
- whether there is a need for further treatment at home or in hospital.

Remember that successful planning and implementation takes some time. Although a patient may be keen to get home and the hospital may desperately need the bed, a rushed discharge is more likely to result in the patient having to be readmitted.

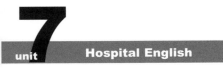

Look at examples of discharge letters that have been written by other members of your team to GPs, district nurses and care agencies. Writing a letter is one of the nurse's most difficult tasks and is particularly time-consuming. Looking at good models can save you time when it is your turn to write a letter!

If you and other members of your team have taken accurate and comprehensive information about your patient from the patient, relatives or close friends and noted information from doctors, occupational therapists and physiotherapists your job will be made so much easier.

Once you have been involved in the transfer or discharge of patients, reflect on what other information, teaching and support might have been useful for you:

I would like to have known......

7.2 Making phone calls

There are various ways of making your telephone English more efficient.
The first step is to notice how your colleagues use the phone, and then try and use the same language yourself.

7.2.a

Below are some examples of what nurses might say on the phone. Match the expressions to the function.

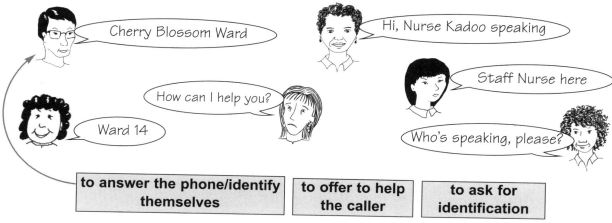

Cherry Blossom Ward

Hi, Nurse Kadoo speaking

How can I help you?

Staff Nurse here

Ward 14

Who's speaking, please?

| to answer the phone/identify themselves | to offer to help the caller | to ask for identification |

7.2.b

What do your colleagues actually say when they are on the phone?
Sit by the phone and write down here the words and expressions you hear.
What do they say …

to explain that a colleague is not available...

to take a message for a colleague..

to ask the other person to repeat what they said..

to ask the other person to clarify what they said...

to confirm information...

to decline giving information...

to respond to thanks..

to say goodbye/sign off..

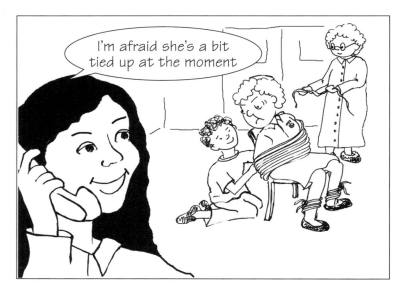

I'm afraid she's a bit tied up at the moment

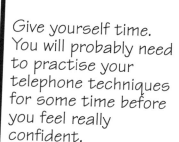

Give yourself time. You will probably need to practise your telephone techniques for some time before you feel really confident.

Of course, all phone calls are different in content, but they usually follow a similar pattern of turn-taking. If you can recognise the pattern, you can begin to guess what the caller is likely to say next. This makes it much easier to communicate.

Notice the pattern

Recognise the pattern the next time

Know what's coming next

Communicate better

7.2.c

Pattern 1 – Making a call

What you are doing	What you say
Greetings	*Hello*
Identify yourself	*This is*
Asking to speak to someone	
Explaining purpose of call	
Showing you understand	
Offering to leave a message	
Thanking	
Ending the call	

7.2.d

Look at these phrases from a telephone conversation. What do you think the reply will be in each case?

1 Can I take a message for him? ....

2 Can I speak to
Staff Nurse Delgado, please? ....

3 Who shall I say is calling? ....

4 Hold on a second. I'll just get her. ....

5 Sorry – did you say s-m-Y-t-h? ....

There could be hundreds of different answers - some suggested answers are in the key!

How do the nurses on your ward reply to these phrases? Try using them and write down the replies. They may be very different from the ones we suggested!

7.2.e

Pattern 2 – Answering a call

What you are doing	What you say
Picking up the phone and identifying yourself	
Helping the caller	
Asking for identification and information	
Explaining that someone is not available	
Suggesting alternative actions	
Confirming	
Declining information	
Responding to thanks	
Signing off	

7.3 Record keeping

Nurses are normally concerned with writing notes for reference purposes to keep up the medical records. However, the NMC state that:

> Healthcare records are a tool of communication within the team.
>
> *NMC Code of Professional Conduct page 6*

They place emphasis on sharing of knowledge for the benefit of the patient. Sharing can only be effective if information gathering and recording is of a high standard.

As you will know in most clinical areas there is not just a single document but many documents which must be maintained, although in some hospitals multidisciplinary documentation is being introduced.

There is a wealth of clear cut advice about the legal aspects of record keeping. Because you need an awareness of laws such as the Human Rights Act 1998 and the Data Protection Act 1998 employers usually familiarise their employees with the essentials in their induction programmes.

Patients are increasingly exercising their rights to access to records and to comment on their treatment. In some instances patients hold their own records. In a legal case your records are a major part of the evidence. 'Under the UK legal system, a patient may bring a case for negligence up to 3 years after the event.' (Watson, 2002, Clinical nursing and related sciences, page 12)

Remember you are accountable for your actions and so need to document them – even where you decided not to take action this should be documented!

The NMC Code of Professional Conduct states that nurses

> must ensure that the healthcare record for the patient or client is, 'an accurate account of treatment, care planning and delivery.'
>
> *NMC Code of Professional Conduct page 6*

The NMC criteria

- Documents should be written as soon as possible after the event has taken place
- If possible the patient should be involved in their completion
- It should show evidence of how care is

    decided upon   planned

    delivered   evaluated

The NMC's comprehensive leaflet Guidelines for Records and Record Keeping (2002) is essential reading.

The next exercises invite you to reflect on the content, accuracy and style of your own record keeping.

7.3.a

Is there any aspect of your written English that could be improved? Tick as necessary.

☐ Accurate English grammar e.g. use of tenses, prepositions

☐ Neat handwriting – is it easy for others to read?

☐ Expressive language – do you ever find yourself searching for the correct word or think that you could have used a more suitable word/phrase?

☐ Too dependent on abbreviations and acronyms? (The NMC say that they should not be used at all)

☐ Spelling

If you are unsure about your self-assessment ask your mentor or *Brilliant* buddy to help you. Perhaps you could write a mock patient report and ask them to help you assess its strengths and weaknesses.

Using your checklist decide on an action plan for improvement. For example:

> *Spelling*
>
> *I will use my dictionary more often. When I put a new word or phrase in my lexicon I will check it when I get home*
>
> *When I'm on the phone I will ask the speaker to spell long words out for me*
>
> *I will use a spell checker on the computer when I type a document, then I'll make a note in my lexicon of the correct spelling*
>
> *I will ask my friends to tell me if I have spelt something wrong*

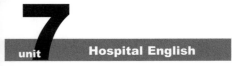

7.3.b

Choose a document with handwritten notes.

Using the checklist below and the NMC's criteria above evaluate the document.

Describe the document.

Does it have the following features?

Legible ☐

In dark permanent ink ☐

Any errors crossed through with a single line, dated and signed ☐

Signed, dated and timed ☐

Factual (not subjective) ☐

Has evidence to back up any decisions ☐

Free from jargon ☐

Free from abbreviations and acronyms ☐

Gives a picture of what the nurse did, heard and observed ☐

Reports actual phrases that were said by a patient or colleague ☐

Refers appropriately to any other documents such as care plan, observation charts etc. ☐

7.4 The legal framework

Caulfield* usefully divides regulation in healthcare into two main branches, 'objective rules' and 'subjective rules'. Subjective rules are social, moral and personal choices made by the nurse. For you, as an international nurse with your own beliefs, values and cultural frameworks, it may be necessary to be sensitive to the accepted norms of the society and culture of the UK as well as reflecting on your own professional standards.

Objective rules are defined as, 'Being imposed, enforced and obligatory and frequently applied to areas of professional work where a clear statement of guidance and control is required for reasons of safety and public policy.' Examples of these are

- Your Code of Professional Conduct
- English (or Scottish) Civil Law (including vicarious liability)
- English (or Scottish) Criminal Law (slightly different in Scotland)
- Accountability to the employer

It may seem a little frightening to be faced with so much new important information. You must understand the seriousness of breaking (or bending) rules or laws – you could be putting your professional registration at risk as well as your patient. But, equally important, you must be appropriately supported by your employer to minimise the risk of breaking the law out of ignorance – because you didn't know better – this is where the emphasis on training days comes from.

In addition there are situations where there are no clear legal guidelines. So exercising your professional judgement is critical! Better still is checking your professional judgement against those of your colleagues – would they understand and agree with your actions?

* Caulfield H. The legal and professional framework of nursing in Balliere's Nurses' Dictionary, Balliere Tindall & RCN, (2002) page 487

Protecting the patient

You may notice in the UK that there is great emphasis on protecting the patient. After all we all pay National Insurance contributions from our wages to receive safe and effective healthcare. The NHS Plan* sets out 'to create a health service designed around the needs of the patients'. In the Professional Code of Conduct there is also central emphasis on accountability and the duty of care to patients.

We hear of horror stories about nurses who made errors at work, but in fact removal from the professional register and being disciplined by an employer happens to very few people. Criminal prosecution is even rarer.

'Near-miss' reporting

Unless a patient dies or suffers serious harm any misconduct is likely to be dealt with internally. If you are working in a hospital, incident reporting should be explained to you during your induction programme. If something in your area nearly goes wrong – but not quite – such as a regular mix up of drugs which have similar packaging – but nothing has yet gone wrong – we call these incidents 'near-misses'. Most employers have a 'near-miss' reporting system to try to build up a pattern of risks which they can then tackle before anything actually goes wrong. If your place of work operates a 'near miss' reporting system or a 'no blame policy', this will help you feel confident in reporting any mistakes. Check with your ward manager if you want to review the procedures for reporting near misses in your area.

Accountability

It's a little frightening to be faced with so much new information and the potential seriousness of breaking the rules or law but you should be appropriately supported by your employer to minimise the risk of doing so. This is why each hospital has its own guidelines, procedures and protocols and why it is so important to learn and follow them.

A nurse might be held in law to account for their actions in

- treating a patient without consent
- failing to provide safe or competent care
- making a drug error
- breaching confidentiality
- being untrustworthy such as, stealing from a patient or employer.

Depending on the seriousness of an event a nurse may be called to account from all four different spheres of law. For example if a patient dies there may be implications for criminal law, civil law, professional conduct committee and the employer.

* The NHS Plan, Dept. of Health, London July 2000, CM4818

Nursing and Midwifery Council Code of Professional Conduct

This a useful small book which clearly sets out the code. It demonstrates how your personal accountability is manifested in your working life. One of the main purposes of the code is to protect the patient or client.

There are other sources to keep you informed of the nurse's position. Nursing journals report serious incidents which you could use as a focus for discussion. The NMC's quarterly publications including the Professional Conduct Annual Report are useful to read as are the RCN and UNISON publications discussing duty of care and rights of the nurse.

If you read or see anything that you don't understand make a note to ask a senior member of staff or consult the website of a professional body.

It is a good idea to become a member of a professional organisation or trade union. These organisations will keep you up to date and protect you if you ever face litigation. Look out for information on your hospital notice-boards.

7.4.a

Read and research.
Can you think of how you might prepare yourself as fully as possible in the UK? Here are a few of our suggestions.

Always keep a reference of what you read or courses you attend.

Read relevant NMC Documents.

Read your job description.

Read your contract of employment.

Read information given to you at your induction programme (this will be mainly policies and procedures).

Read Health and Safety notices and publications.

Read professional guidelines written by the Royal College of Nursing or Unison (both have specific information aimed at international nurses).

Become a member of a professional organisation or trade union such as Unison or the Royal College of Nursing, to keep you up to date and to protect you if you face litigation. Look out for information on your hospital noticeboards.

Make a note of things you don't fully understand and ask a senior member of staff or consult the website of a professional body. It is no excuse to say you didn't know that a regulation, policy or law existed!

www.rcn.org.uk   www.nmc-uk.org   www.unison.org.uk   www.doh.gov.uk

UNIT 7   Assignment

Transfer of care in your hospital

Research and write out the procedures which govern how patients are discharged or transferred from your area. If you complete the four tasks below you will have completed the assignment.

> You may find it helpful to spend time with the hospital Discharge Co-ordinator, to attend interdisciplinary meetings and ideally to spend extra time looking at patient notes and at documentation that may have been written on previous discharges or transfers.

Task 1

Write out a list of people or departments that you may have to consult to arrange a patient discharge.

Task 2

Your job is to give as full a picture as possible of the patient including:

- their past medical history

- their treatment and care in hospital

- their current physical, mental and emotional state

- where they live and with whom

- what type of accommodation the patient has

- what other agencies and services have previously been involved

- whether there is a need for further treatment at home or in hospital.

Make a list under each the above headings of some questions you might ask to obtain information.

Task 3

Find and read the relevant policies which govern discharge planning and discuss these with an experienced nurse.

Study typical letters to external agencies. Note some of the language used to describe the patients' needs and how any requests are made.

Task 4

Evaluate the procedures that you have researched. Consider:

- ease of access to support for the nurse and for the patient

- how fully the procedures are implemented

- how much paperwork is involved

- if there are areas of discharge planning which could be improved

- how the discharge planning process compares to your previous hospital experience.

Learning Objectives

On completion of this assignment you will be able to:

- describe the procedures and policies governing transfer or discharge of your patients to your mentor

- explain the procedures of transfer or discharge to your patient

- know who to contact regarding discharge/transfer

- know what the challenges are in your area to discharging patients

- know what a model letter to an external agency looks like

- ask relevant questions to gather information you might need.

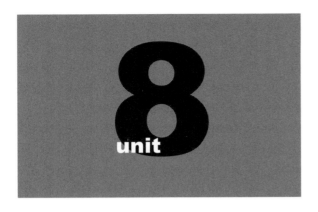

Infection control

Communication while giving personal care

Did you get a sample?
Slang on the loo
Present your talk

Your competency framework

Assess your language and communication skills and make an action plan

8.1   Infection control

All healthcare workers need to know how to control the spread of infection.

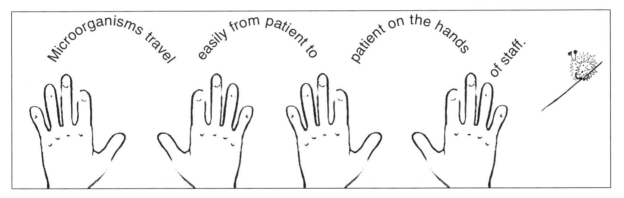

Microorganisms travel easily from patient to patient on the hands of staff.

However it is hard to measure the results of good infection control practices because, unlike more obvious aspects of care, with infection control you are more likely to see the results of a lack of control than where control has been successfully exercised. The government is interested in new ways of measuring effective infection control and some types, such as MRSA, are recorded for statistical purposes. ◄———

> What does MRSA stand for? Are there any other infections you regularly look out for in your area?

Infection control is an area to keep constantly under review starting with which infections are predominant in your area and how they are transmitted. Nurses need to look at the occurrence or epidemiology of the population with whom they are working as well as at the control of nosocomial (hospital acquired) infections. We are aiming to protect our patients and protect ourselves. During your workplace induction you should be given a summary of prevalent infections and of the key infection control ◄——— measures.

> Were you given this information? Where is it now? How well do you remember the key control measures?

Universal precautions

Universal precautions will be familiar to you but it is good to try to recall them. This way you can ensure that you are aware of any differences in names of equipment or procedures. You may be used to different practices in your previous workplace - check if they are the same here (e.g. use of face masks).

8.1.a

Here is a list of some universal precautions. Add any basic information you know and note how this compares to your previous workplace.

My hospital procedure and notes

Handwashing

Cuts and abrasions

Gloves

Needlestick injury

Waste disposal

Aprons

Eye protection

Spillages/disinfection

Patient communication

A patient who does not understand that these precautions are routine may feel anxious. They may think that they are getting special treatment.

8.1.b

Match the reassurance and explanations below to your actions.

What you do   **What you say to the patient**

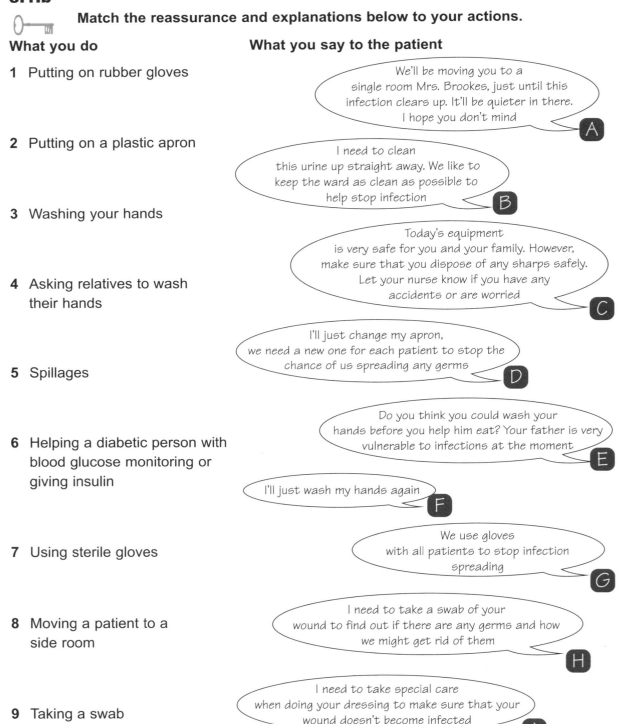

1 Putting on rubber gloves

2 Putting on a plastic apron

3 Washing your hands

4 Asking relatives to wash their hands

5 Spillages

6 Helping a diabetic person with blood glucose monitoring or giving insulin

7 Using sterile gloves

8 Moving a patient to a side room

9 Taking a swab

150

8.2 Communication while giving personal care

For a UK nurse helping a patient with personal care such as washing, elimination and eating can be a main part of their daily duties. In your previous workplace many of these activities might have been the responsibility of a patient's relatives. In addition in U.K. hospitals there is a growing elderly population. Although nursing places emphasis on maintaining or restoring the independence of the elderly person you are likely to have many elderly patients who need your help.

Even if your physical skills in helping someone with their personal care are excellent it may take some time and effort to become competent in communicating with the patient whilst you are working. Doing and talking at the same time can be difficult! As well as being good for building a friendly relationship effective communication is an important part of establishing the patient's consent to your actions.

As an international nurse you are developing your communication and clinical skills at speed in an intensive environment. Helping with personal care gives you the perfect opportunity to do both.

8.2.a

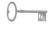 **Arrange to observe another nurse carrying out some aspect of personal care. (If this is not possible, recall a patient that you have recently cared for.)**

Remember you should get the consent of the patient before starting the observation. Note down the language you hear used by the nurse and the replies given by the patient. List the sort of phrases you hear the other nurses use. If you have a *Brilliant* buddy you can share your experiences of personal care and build up your vocabulary.

Hair care

Mouth care

Here is an example of the sort of language you might use while washing a patient.

> Would you like a shower today? I can help you as much as you want

> You said you didn't sleep well, would you like a bit more help this morning or can you manage?

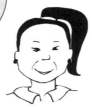

> Good morning Mrs Biggs, I'm going to help you have a wash. What shall we do today, shower, bath or an all over wash by the bed?

> If you have a wash in the chair I could help you with the bits that you can't reach. Is that alright?

> If you sit at the basin and do what you can. Press the buzzer and I'll help you with the rest. Is that OK?

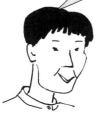

As you wash someone or groom someone's hair it is usual to chat. This can be therapeutically useful as you can find out how your patient is psychologically responding to their treatment. However, even if your patient is very tired and may not feel like responding, words that reassure or encourage can still be used.

Notice that while you are offering help and encouraging the patient to do as much for themselves as possible (to foster independence) you are constantly checking with the patient that they are happy - and therefore you are gaining consent.

Respect your patient's privacy and dignity at all times by offering choices and by assuring privacy, such as checking that they are not overlooked during a wash.

Listening is an important part of communication.

It is helpful to the team to make a note of or pass on to senior staff any relevant information that your patient tells you while you are with them. You and your team may need to decide whether action needs to be taken to resolve any issues that your patient had on their mind.

8.2.b

Here are some phrases used by nurses – can you guess the context?
Where are they and what are they doing?

Listen and collect at least three more phrases in My Personal Lexicon.

a *How's that water temperature?*

b *Do you like soap or shower gel?*

c *Shall I wash your back now?*

d *Tell me if that's uncomfortable.*

e *Is that OK?*

f *Tell me when you've had enough.*

g *Tell me if I press too hard.*

h *Shall I wash down below for you?
(genital area)*

i *Would you like to do that yourself?*

8.2.c

These are the sort of questions you might ask your patient.
Suggest some typical replies

a How did you sleep last night?

b Are you expecting any visitors today?

c Did you have much breakfast?

d How are you managing to move around?

e Is your pain relief working?

f How are you feeling about....?

g Has your leg/back/stomach been giving you any more trouble?

h Have you had any more problems with indigestion?

8.3   Did you get a sample?

Test yourself

If a patient said this to you, would you know what they meant?

1 'I've just been for a wee, nurse, and it hurts like hell!'

2 'Excuse me, dear, I need to do number twos…'

3 'Can I have a bottle please, Sandra?'

If you don't know, look at Maria's Lexicon on page 159.

Talking to patients about using the toilet is one of the most potentially confusing communications you can have. There are lots of slang expressions associated with using the toilet and naturally, patients are often embarrassed to say what they actually mean. So they use a special phrase or euphemism which may be in the local dialect or even just a phrase used in their own family.

And of course, if verbal communication breaks down, it's much more difficult to explain using mime!

We have divided the topic into two areas:

- clinical language (focusing on the stool chart)
- patient-related language (focusing on slang and euphemism).

> Interesting fact: the word lavatory, which is now a very common British English word for the toilet, was originally itself a euphemism. (It meant a place where you wash.) Now people use other expressions so they don't have to say lavatory!

The stool chart

Most wards and hospitals will use a stool chart, although the actual format of the chart may differ. Below, we show you a typical one from a UK hospital, but before you look at it, think about the following questions:

8.3.a

1   What's a stool chart for?

2   In your experience, what kind of information is entered on a stool chart?

3   In hospitals where you have worked, who was allowed to see it?

Now look at a typical UK example, and say in what ways it differs from stool charts you have known.

STOOL CHART			SURNAME FIRST NAMES			
DATE	TIME	COLOUR	CONSISTENCY	WEIGHT	HAEM- +OCCULT-	OTHER COMMENTS

8.3.b

Here is some more language which you might come across in the stool charts. In which columns would you put the expressions in the grey box?

> yellowy   offensive   greenish   watery
> mucousy   dark brown   loose   semi-formed

To learn the kinds of expressions and entries that your colleagues would write on the stool chart in your area, find a time to do some research.

8.3.c

Collect a number, say 10, completed stool charts on your ward.
Now observe what your experienced colleagues write in each column of the stool chart.
If you want to, make a list in My Personal Lexicon of typical language used.
This may help you find the right language when you need it.

This language is normally medically or clinically based and therefore not suitable for using in talking to patients. One of your tasks is to suit the language to the person you are speaking to. In general, avoiding clinical jargon or medical terms is sensible – that's why you need to be familiar with the slang and euphemisms too!

155

8.4 Slang on the loo

Slang and euphemism are used very widely by British people when talking about going to the toilet. This avoidance of saying what we mean results in a wide variety of obscure expressions learnt from childhood. In stressful circumstances, such as being in hospital, it is not unusual for people to resort to child language because they are embarrassed about bodily functions.

Another complication is that culturally the strongest words for toilet-going are also used as the rudest ones for attacking other people! So many words have a dual cultural connotation being both embarrassing and offensive. This makes it very difficult to learn how to use this language in an appropriate and professional way.

In fact, it is very difficult to think of toilet words and expressions in English which are neutral – they are either found in medical/clinical language (like *stool*) or slang/child language (like *poo* or *crap* or *shit*). Our advice is to become familiar with as much of this language as you need – writing it down in My Personal Lexicon and checking its use and meaning – but to speak only the language you feel comfortable with. Your potential vocabulary will grow in this area and your confidence in using the right word in the right place will develop as you notice how others you respect use the language.

8.4.a

 Put the following words and expressions into three groups – ask around if you need help from native speakers

a medical or formal language
b adult slang
c child language

Mark them a, b, or c in the box

my sit-upon ☐

wee-wee ☐

go for a slash ☐

use the washroom ☐

faeces ☐

urinate ☐

number ones ☐

stool ☐

piss ☐

In fact, even within these groupings, there are differences. Just as we can make a distinction between medical and non-medical language so we can talk about the difference between formal and informal use of language. Slang being a type of informal language normally used in an informal context.

So you can see from the position of the words on the chart below that *stool* is in the top right quarter, because it is used in a formal medical context whereas *go for a slash* is slang and non-medical.

Native speakers of English will move between these different quadrants depending on their situation and who they are speaking to.

8.4.b

Put the words and phrases from Maria's lexicon on page 159 into the correct quadrant of the chart.

medical

stool

informal eg slang   **formal**

go for a slash

non-medical

1
Become sensitive to fine cultural distinctions between words. If you are not sure, ask! These distinctions are important because they might help you to decide which language to use with whom.

2
Sometimes, especially with children, there is a special word used only in that family and nowhere else! We have heard of a family which used the phrase 'doing a gruntie' to mean 'producing faeces' but nobody else in southern England ever knew what they were talking about.

3
Often different regions of Britain have different words. (This is true of other topics like food and drink and clothes.) Make sure you notice the words from the region where you work, as well as more general ones.

8.4.c

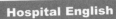 **Now look at the dialogue between a nurse and a patient, and fill in the gaps with words and expressions from the chart. How would you finish the nurse's last speech?**

Patient   Nurse, I need to ....

Nurse   OK, Mr Severn, I'll bring you a ....

Patient   Ta.

Nurse   Have you .... already today?

Patient   No. In fact, I'm a bit worried about it. Usually my .... are fine, but since I've been in hospital…

Nurse   Oh, don't worry, Mr Severn, it's quite normal.

Patient   And the other thing is that when I ...., my, you know, my

.... is a bit of a funny colour.

Nurse   I see. And when did you first notice this?

Patient   Yesterday evening.

Nurse   Well, I'll mention it to the doctor, and we might need an ....

Patient   A what?

Nurse   Sorry, Mr Severn, that means a midstream urine specimen …

Colloquial English is rich in toilet talk and you may find colleagues and patients will love telling you about their favourite words. Collect the language in a separate section of My Personal Lexicon. On page 159 is a page from Maria's lexicon

8.4.d

Look at the collection of language taken from Maria's Personal Lexicon, and see how many of the expressions are:

a already familiar

b new to you.

> Remember – you need to know what these words mean but you don't need to use them yourself unless you feel comfortable doing so.

158

Slang on the loo in Maria's Personal Lexicon

WORD/PHRASE/ABBREVIATION	MEANING	EXAMPLES/NOTES
1 to pee/wee/ spend a penny	To urinate	I need a wee/I want to spend a penny
2 waterworks	Bladder and associated organs	I've got waterworks trouble
3 going for a slash/piss going to see a man about a dog	Going to the toilet	Slang, mainly used by men
4 Have you passed water today?	Have you urinated today?	Polite, used to patients
5 wet myself/pissed my pants	Wet clothes/bed, usually accident	I'm really sorry, but I've wet myself
6 have a poo/shit/ crap/number two	Had bowels open	I can't poo on hospital toilets
7 bunged up	Constipated	I've been really bunged up since my op. (operation)
8 dying for the loo bursting for a pee	Desperate to urinate	Quick! I'm bursting for a pee
9 bottle	Portable urinal	Leave a bottle at the side of my bed, will ya, nurse?'
10 potty	Child's portable toilet	Look, mummy, I've done a wee-wee in my potty
11 commode	Toilet that can be wheeled to patient's bedside	Nurse! Quick, I need the commode
12 the runs	Diarrhoea	He had the runs for three days
13 backside/bum/arse	Bottom	I get an itchy bum at night
14 sluice	Storage area for bedpans etc and disposal/dirty area	Chuck it in the sluice, will 'ya?
15 BNO	Bowels not open	Abbreviation used on chart
16 MSU	Midstream urine specimen	Common abbreviation
17 pants/knickers/ drawers/smalls/ undies (female)/ shorts/underpants/ boxers (male)	Lower undergarments/ underwear	'ere, love, give us a hand with my undies, will 'ya?
18 HNPU	Has not passed urine	Abbreviation used on chart
19 bog/loo paper	Toilet roll	There's no bog paper in this loo
20. caught short	Desperately needing to urinate when in a public place	I was caught short in the market

8.5   Your competency framework

If you are in a period of adaptation or induction you will have been given a list of the competencies which you are expected to complete before you can submit your papers for registration.

You will have a mentor or supervisor who will help you gather the evidence to show you have achieved each of the competencies. However, it is your responsibility to keep an accurate record of how and when you have reached your goals.

Here are some of the methods used to assess competence.

1 Observation of practice and documentation.

2 Written or verbal questioning.

3 Self-report validated by witness.

4 Simulation.

Here are some examples of competency statements.

a Demonstrate an understanding of the main elements of Standards of Record Keeping (NMC) and apply this in practice.

b Function effectively in a team and participate in a multi-professional approach to the care of patients.

c Implement the planned programme of care and effectively manage a caseload of patients.

Negotiating

As you work with your mentor you may need to negotiate on a number of points. This is where you put forward a suggestion and discuss a solution which suits you and your mentor.

You may need to discuss:

- what evidence is appropriate for a particular competency
- what else needs to be done to fulfil the competency framework
- if a competency statement seems particularly complex, could it be broken down into smaller parts?
- you may need longer to complete a competency (or your mentor may suggest that you are not ready)– ask for the time
- you may feel that the evidence has been submitted (or the competency has been demonstrated) already but not signed off – describe what has happened and ask for it to be sorted out
- you may need to spend some time in a different setting, if you are in theatres or ICU for example, because some elements of the competency framework may be difficult to demonstrate. Ask for this to be arranged for you.

What language could you use to negotiate?

Polite suggestion

Would it be possible to ...

I'd like to see if...

Next time I think I should...

I don't think I'm quite ready to...

I think I'm ready to...

Asking for your supervisor's view

What do you think?

What's your thinking on that one?

Do you think that's fair?

Do you agree?

Time management

Could you find time to...

If I come in early next week, could we go over...

When do you think we'll be able to...

Could we make a deadline for...

This week I would like to complete...

8.5.a

Choose one competency statement.

Decide which method is appropriate to use to prove your competence.

Imagine you are going to meet your mentor for a review meeting. Prepare your evidence or questions.

Rehearse the meeting with your *Brilliant* buddy. You can be the nurse and your buddy the mentor. Explain your position. Discuss the matter briefly and negotiate a solution. Now swap roles.

With the competency framework we find that nurses who take charge of the process of completing it do much better than those who wait for the mentor to drive it along! Be active and take charge!

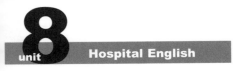

8.6   Present your talk

If you are working in a class choose a time this week to present the talk which you prepared as Assignment 5.

If you are working with your *Brilliant* buddy plan when and where you can meet, perhaps with some more friends, to give this talk.

When giving your talk

Introduce yourself

Use notes on card and address your audience directly

Use eye contact and smile

Do not read from your notes, present them confidently

Ask for questions at the end

Keep to the time limit — maximum 5 minutes

When listening to a talk

It is customary to be silent when watching a talk

Take notes if you want to

Be ready to ask questions

Afterwards celebrate your achievement! It takes courage to stand up and address people so you have already done *Brilliantly*!

Feedback

When you feel ready, ask for some feedback on your performance. Here are some criteria you could use.

Communication
- Could your audience follow your talk?
- Clear expression, structure and verbal sign-posting.

Content
- Was it relevant and up to date information?
- What sources did you use? Did you summarise and analyse the data appropriately?

Speaking and listening skills
- Were you easy to understand (intelligible)?
- Could you answer questions on the spot effectively?

UNIT 8 Assignment

Assess your language and communication skills and propose an action plan for continuing learning

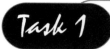 *Task 1* **Self-assess your language skills.**

We are going to divide language skills into five areas
- listening
- reading
- speaking – interaction (talking with other people, both socially and professionally)
- speaking - production (describing, telling stories, presenting)
- writing.

1 Which ones are most important for you? Give each area a score out of ten for its importance to you. Ten is very important, while zero is not important at all. We are talking about both at work and socially. Write the score in **Box A**.

2 Now look at the self-assessment grid on p175 and for each of the five areas above, decide which of the four descriptions B1, B2, C1 or C2 is the closest to a description of your ability in that area. Put this description in **Box B**.

3 Now, in **Box C**, if you choose B1 give yourself 5 points, B2 10 points, C1 15 points and C2 20 points.

4 Now for each skill, multiply the score in Box A by your self-assessment score in Box C. This will give you an achievement score for that area in Box D.

For example if you think writing is very important you might give yourself 9 in Box A. If you think your level for writing on the grid is B2, your self-assessment score will be 10 and so your achievement score will be 90 (9x10).

Area	A Importance to me score	B From grid on page 175	C Points	D Achievement score
Listening				
Reading				
Speaking – interaction				
Speaking – production				
Writing				

163

Results

If you have a high score (**between 170 and 200**), this shows that this area is important for you, and that you are good at it.
You don't need to do anything at this point!

If you have a low score, (**below 50**), this shows that you are not very happy with your performance in this area, but that in any case it is not a high priority for you.
You don't need to do anything about this area at the present time, but you might need to if you decided to improve your skills.

If you have medium score, (**between 50 and 170**) this means either you are not happy with your performance, or this is an important area for you, or both.
These are the areas you need to work on.

Task 2 — Assess your communication skills.
Consider how far you have improved your communication skills and confidence in using them in the workplace

On the scale below assess how much you agree with the following statements?

5	4	3	2	1
completely agree	mostly agree	no particular opinion	disagree	no change noticed

What I have practised during this communication skills course	5	4	3	2	1
… has contributed to my personal development					
… has helped me develop and maintain my professional relationships					
… has helped me share information with my colleagues and patients					
… has helped me to maintain and develop a sense of self-confidence and self-worth					
… has helped me learn how to find new information from a variety of sources					
… has improved my standard English pronunciation					
… has developed my confidence in choosing the appropriate communication strategy needed to enhance my own nursing practice					

Task 3

Summarise the information you have collected and write a report about your own language and communication skills.

This should be written in as objective a way as possible using the following structure:

1 describe your findings

2 analyse the findings

3 draw conclusions and suggest action for the future.

The action plan should include which areas need work and some suggestions as to how you might improve them. If you are stuck for ideas for the latter, we have a checklist for each area on page 176.

Learning Objectives

After this assignment you will be able to:

- reflecte on your progress
- describe your strengths in language skills
- describe your strengths in communication skills
- plan any action you need for continuing learning to address your needs.

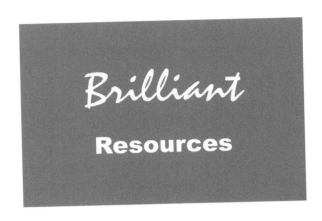

Resources

Building My *Brilliant* Portfolio

You can start now to build up a collection of your working papers into a tidy and organised folder.

A ring binder is a good place to keep pages organised.

Call this folder My *Brilliant* Portfolio

Keep your Hospital English assignments in the portfolio.

For My *Brilliant* Portfolio here are some other things you might collect in your ring binder:

- leaflets for patients in your area
- published articles useful to you in extending your clinical knowledge
- copies of procedures and policies you have been given
- assignments and rough drafts of work
- examples of professional documents including letters
- certificates of courses completed
- reflective writing.

Can you add some more things?

> As a Registered Nurse you will need to keep a similar folder in your professional life according to a standard laid down by the NMC. It is called your record of Post-Registration Education and Practice (PREP). For more information about this see The PREP Handbook published by the Nursing and Midwifery Council.
>
> 6.1 You must keep your knowledge and skills up-to-date throughout your working life. In particular, you should take part regularly in learning activities that develop your competence and performance
>
> *NMC Code of Professional Conduct page 8*

Working with a *Brilliant* buddy

A self-study programme is difficult to undertake by yourself. It can be easy to start with good intentions and then stop because you do not make the time or you lose heart. For encouragement and motivation look for a *Brilliant* buddy!

Why not find another international nurse who might be happy to follow the programme with you?

Finding a buddy

- Ask another nurse in your unit.
- Ask one of the Professional Development Nurses if they know anyone in a different unit who might be interested.
- Ask your International Officer in the Human Resources department if they know of any new international arrivals.

Start a buddy system

You may have a Mentor and Deputy Mentor chosen for you by the hospital in which you are working. Their role is to help you to be successful in meeting your clinical competency objectives.

A buddy system, on the other hand, is where someone like you, a co-worker or colleague, works with you to continue to reflect on your practice. You help your buddy and your buddy helps you.

R.1.a

Think about what role a buddy can play?

R.1.b

What is the value of a buddy system?

What are the ground rules for being someone's buddy? How should you both behave?

Ground rules are the basic rules which you agree on before you start to work together. They can govern simple things such as agreeing how much notice you need to give if you are going to cancel a meeting, or complex things, such as deciding what is the appropriate level of confidentiality to adopt.

When to meet

Meet regularly for a length of time that is realistic and feasible for both of you, say every Wednesday for half an hour.

Where to meet

Find a quiet place where you feel safe and where you won't get interrupted, preferably not your bedroom or the nurses' staffroom! A corner of a quiet canteen might do.

Agreements

Establish whatever agreements you want for safety and efficiency e.g. starting and stopping meetings on time, maintaining confidentiality, encouraging each other to express your feelings as well as your thoughts.

What to talk about

Decide on a topic in advance so you do not waste time when you meet. This should be related to your professional life rather than your social life!

Balance

Mark Twain said 'It's a terrible death to be talked to death' so ensure that both of you get time to talk and share your experiences.

HELP
Could you be My Buddy?

I am an international nurse

from ....

working at .... hospital.

I am studying the Arakelian Hospital English: communication programme to improve my language and communication skills and give me more confidence.

I am looking for another nurse to work with me for a month as my Buddy, meeting once a week at the hospital.

If you are interested get in touch with

....

Nurse: ....

Photocopiable © 2003 Arakelian Programmes 01865 849768

Hospital English: the Brilliant learning workbook for international nurses

Brilliant buddy worksheet

Name...Contact...

Agree with your buddy before the first meeting:

1 Where are you going to meet

....

2 When

....

3 For how long

....

At your first meeting:

1 Agree the ground rules

....

....

2 Think about your role as a buddy

• One thing I feel good about

....

• One thing I don't feel confident about

....

• What I would like to discuss next week

....

169

Making a *Brilliant* Call

Asking for somebody

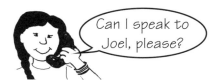

Can I speak to Joel, please?

Leaving a message

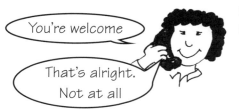

Could you get him to ring me back?

Could you take a message?

Asking for a department

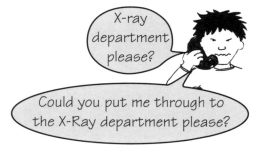

X-ray department please?

Could you put me through to the X-Ray department please?

Apologetic /difficult requests

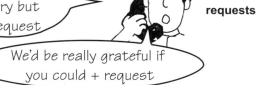

I'm dreadfully sorry but + request

We'd be really grateful if you could + request

Checking who you are speaking to

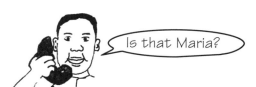

Is that Maria?

Checking details

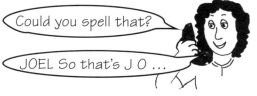

Can I just check the details again?

Can I just check that?

Explaining purpose of a call

We have a problem with …

It's about a patient who has …

We have a patient who needs …

It's regarding …

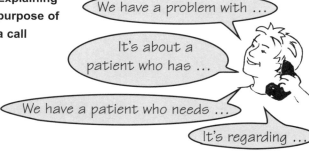

Checking spelling

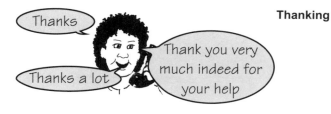

Could you spell that?

JOEL So that's J O …

Thanking

Thanks

Thanks a lot

Thank you very much indeed for your help

Asking for information

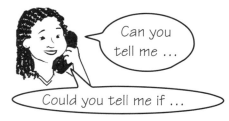

Can you tell me …

Could you tell me if …

Examples: Could you tell me where he lives?
Can you tell me why the operation has been postponed?
Can you tell me if the patient has been admitted?

Responding to thanks

You're welcome

That's alright. Not at all

Photocopiable © 2003 Arakelian Programmes 01865 849768

Hospital English: the Brilliant learning workbook for international nurses

Taking a *Brilliant* Call

Answering the phone

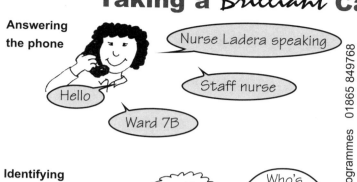

Nurse Ladera speaking

Staff nurse

Hello

Ward 7B

Asking somebody to ring back later

Could you ring back later?

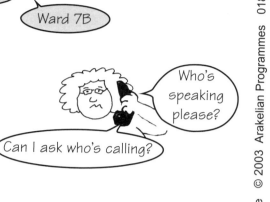

Identifying the caller

Who's speaking please?

Can I ask who's calling?

Suggesting a time to ring back

(Why don't you) Try at 6 o'clock this evening

(Why don't you) Try in about 10 minutes

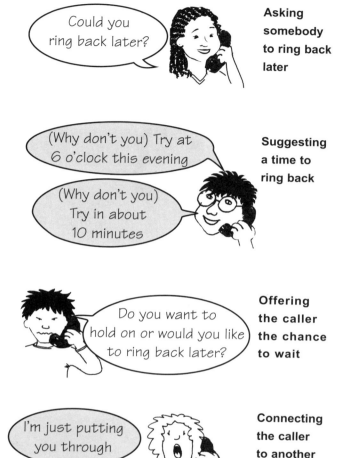

Saying somebody's not here

I'm afraid she's not here at present

She's not around at the moment

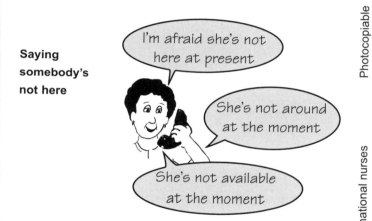

She's not available at the moment

Offering the caller the chance to wait

Do you want to hold on or would you like to ring back later?

Connecting the caller to another phone

I'm just putting you through

I'm just trying to transfer you

I'm just connecting you

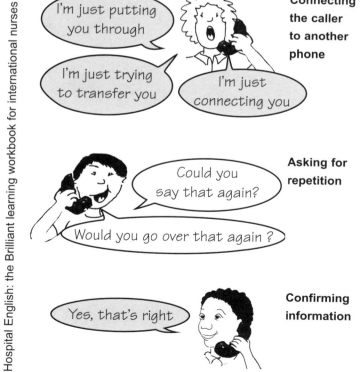

Asking somebody to wait

Sorry to keep you

Just bear with me

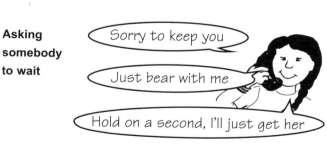

Hold on a second, I'll just get her

Asking for repetition

Could you say that again?

Would you go over that again?

Refusing information

I'm sorry, I'm not allowed to give out that information

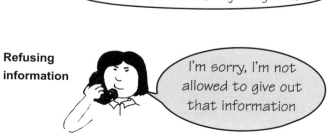

Confirming information

Yes, that's right

Photocopiable © 2003 Arakelian Programmes 01865 849768

Hospital English: the Brilliant learning workbook for international nurses

Pilot's alphabet

On the telephone, it is often difficult to make yourself understood when you are spelling names. This could be because the line is a poor one, or because your pronunication is tricky for the other person! The 'pilot's alphabet' underneath will help you to spell out words correctly – and you can also use it for checking when you don't understand.

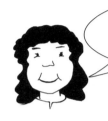

My name is Zoe
that's spelt Z for ZULU,
O for OSCAR, E for ECHO

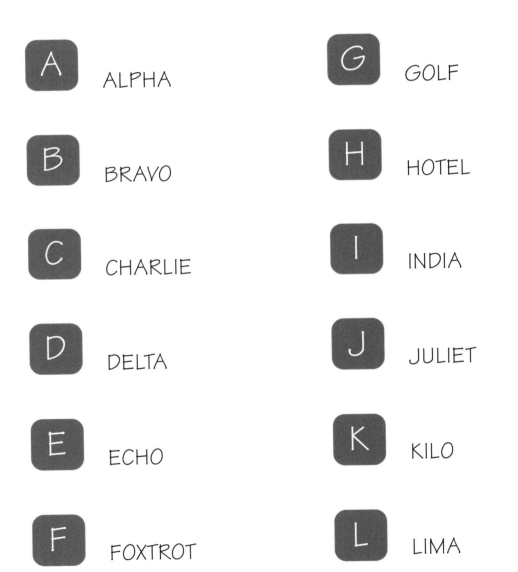

A	ALPHA	
B	BRAVO	
C	CHARLIE	
D	DELTA	
E	ECHO	
F	FOXTROT	
G	GOLF	
H	HOTEL	
I	INDIA	
J	JULIET	
K	KILO	
L	LIMA	

01865 849768

Photocopiable © 2003 Arakelian Programmes

Hospital English: the Brilliant learning workbook for international nurses

Photocopiable © 2003 Arakelian Programmes 01865 849768

Hospital English: the Brilliant learning workbook for international nurses

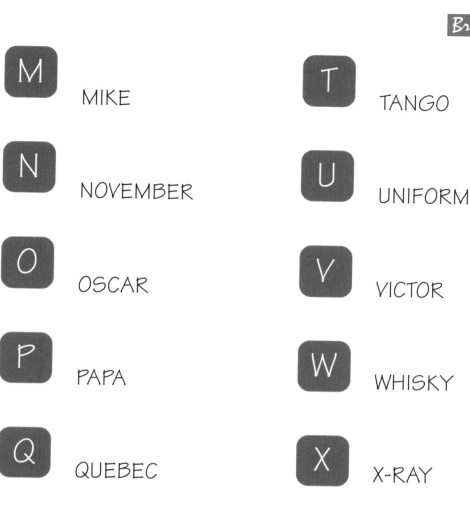

M — MIKE

N — NOVEMBER

O — OSCAR

P — PAPA

Q — QUEBEC

R — ROMEO

S — SIERRA

T — TANGO

U — UNIFORM

V — VICTOR

W — WHISKY

X — X-RAY

Y — YANKEE

Z — ZULU

Make sure you can pronounce the words correctly. Ask a colleague to say them for you, or check in a good dictionary.

Keep this alphabet close to the phone!

173

Self-assessment

You cannot pass or fail this programme, but if you want to track your progress you can use some of the assessment tools described here.

This programme relates to the Common European Framework of Reference for Languages and to the UK National Framework Key Skills specifications for Communication Skills from Level 2 to 4 and ESOL specifications Level 2.

What I can already do

This is a language-centred assessment. Language knowledge is only one part of communication. Your communication skills may be better than your language skills!

Self-assessment grid

Have a look at the 'I can' statements on page 175. Tick the box which most closely matches your own competence in each of these areas.

You will probably find you are at different levels for different skills. This is perfectly normal.

skill \ level	B1	B2	C1	C2
Understanding — listening	I can understand the main points of clear standard speech on familiar matters regularly encountered in work, school, leisure, etc. I can understand the main point of many radio or TV programmes on current affairs or topics of personal or professional interest when the delivery is relatively slow and clear.	I can understand extended speech and lectures and follow even complex lines of argument provided the topic is reasonably familiar. I can understand most TV news and current affairs programmes. I can understand the majority of films in standard dialect.	I can understand extended speech even when it is not clearly structured and when relationships are only implied and not signalled explicitly. I can understand television programmes and films without too much effort.	I have no difficulty in understanding any kind of spoken language, whether live or broadcast, even when delivered at fast native speed, provided I have some time to get familiar with the accent.
Understanding — reading	I can understand texts that consist mainly of high frequency everyday or job-related language. I can understand the description of events, feelings and wishes in personal letters.	I can read articles and reports concerned with contemporary problems in which the writers adopt particular attitudes or viewpoints. I can understand contemporary literary prose.	I can understand long and complex factual and literary texts, appreciating distinctions of style. I can understand specialised articles and longer technical instructions, even when they do not relate to my field.	I can read with ease virtually all forms of the written language, including abstract, structurally or linguistically complex texts such as manuals, specialised articles and literary works.
Speaking — spoken interaction	I can deal with most situations likely to arise whilst travelling in an area where the language is spoken. I can enter unprepared into conversation on topics that are familiar, of personal interest or pertinent to everyday life (e.g. family, hobbies, work, travel and current events).	I can interact with a degree of fluency and spontaneity that makes regular interaction with native speakers quite possible. I can take active part in discussion in familiar contexts, accounting for and sustaining my views.	I can express myself fluently and spontaneously without much obvious searching for expressions. I can use language flexibly and effectively for social and professional purposes. I can formulate ideas and opinions with precision and relate my contribution skilfully to those of other speakers.	I can take part effortlessly in any conversation or discussion and have a good familiarity with idiomatic expressions and colloquialisms. I can express myself fluently and convey finer shades of meaning precisely. If I do have a problem I can backtrack and restructure around the difficulty so smoothly that other people are hardly aware of it.
Speaking — spoken production	I can connect phrases in a simple way in order to describe experiences and events, my dreams, hopes and ambitions. I can briefly give reasons and explanations for opinions and plans. I can narrate a story or relate the plot of a book or film and describe my reactions.	I can present clear, detailed descriptions on a wide range of subjects related to my field of interest. I can explain a viewpoint on a topical issue giving the advantages and disadvantages of various options.	I can present clear, detailed descriptions of complex subjects integrating sub-themes, developing particular points and rounding off with an appropriate conclusion.	I can present a clear, smoothly-flowing description or argument in a style appropriate to the context and with an effective logical structure which helps the recipient to notice and remember significant points.
Writing	I can write simple connected text on topics which are familiar or of personal interest. I can write personal letters describing experiences and impressions.	I can write clear, detailed text on a wide range of subjects relating to my interests. I can write an essay or report, passing on information or giving reasons in support of or against a particular point of view. I can write letters highlighting the personal significance of events and experiences.	I can express myself in clear, well-structured text, expressing points of view at some length. I can write about complex subjects in a letter, an essay or a report, understanding what I consider to be the salient issues. I can select a style appropriate to the reader in mind.	I can write clear, smoothly-flowing text in an appropriate style. I can write complex letters, reports or articles which present a case with effective logical structure which helps the recipient to notice and remember significant points. I can write summaries and reviews of professional or literary works.

Language Self-Assessment Grid from the European Language Portfolio Accredited Model No 9.2001 © 2002 LNTO www.languagesnto.org.uk

Strategies for learning by yourself

Here are some ideas for you to continue to develop your language and communication skills after the programme. You can choose which ones you think will suit you and write them into your action plan in Assignment 8.

Listening

Listen to TV broadcasts or radio programmes for the general meaning.

Choose a radio programme and listen to part of it intensively by trying to write down what you hear and then filling in the missing gaps when you read it again. (If you do this by listening to BBC Radio on the internet you can hear all the articles repeated in the archive section).

Find an English friend for conversation practice.

Try micro-dictations from conversations - listen and write down every word of short bursts of real speech. This is a good technique for trying to build up your telephoning skills – position yourself near the telephone and write down one side of the conversation. Try to guess the other side.

Try listening for key words in repeated situations such as handover, case meetings.

Reading

Borrow or buy graded readers – these are shorter and simpler versions of classic books available in the English Language section of most big bookshops.

Read a graded reader and watch the film at the same time.

Read for up to 30 minutes every day – choose texts you enjoy as well as ones which are 'good for you' and write quick notes summarising the reading.

Form a reading club with some other nurses – you all have to read the same book, or article and then meet up to discuss it (this forces you to read it!)

Don't use a dictionary – it's much more fun and useful to guess meaning.

Speaking – interaction

Go to the pub with friends and agree beforehand to speak only English (or invite an English speaker along to encourage you).

Get a television and watch British TV soaps such as 'Eastenders' as well as the news.

Continue to write down useful expressions in My Personal Lexicon to build up your vocabulary and discuss them with friends.

Speaking – production

Give a running commentary on while you work describing your actions and the thinking processes behind your actions. For example, 'Now I'm going to... this is because I need to check the... '

Practise telling anecdotes to your *Brilliant* buddy.

Report back to your team on professional seminars you have attended.

Writing

Keep a professional diary in My Professional Identity Notebook.

Keep a personal diary or write letters to your friends.

Keep professional letters in a folder for reference, correspondence from a bank for example, so you can use the phrases in your own professional letters.

Keep a record of useful phrases you come across in your own reading, especially in letters and reports – expressions like *I'm looking forward to hearing from you, I'm writing with reference to...*

Communication

Spend your tea breaks in the staff room with others.

Try to get to know new members of the team and offer to help them.

Keep a note of successful encounters you are part of or you see in who/what/where form.

Try to attend social gatherings and professional seminars.

Try to take part in seminars by giving your own opinion.

Let people know how you are getting on and give feedback to your team.

Keep up with your *Brilliant* buddy!

Not all these techniques will work for everybody. Choose what you feel comfortable with.

Keys to exercises

Unit 1

1.1.a

1 N 2 F 3 N 4 P 5 N 6 P (or F) 7 F

1.1.b

1 make a mistake
2 do very well
3 have a listen to your chest
4 get a CT-scan done
5 give somebody the option to do something
6 do the cleaning
7 sound fine
8 have a good time
   also possible have a CT-scan done

1.1.c

1 both 2 both 3 HE 4 HE 5 both 6 both 7 both 8 EE

1.2.a   with our comments

1 b you must carry it with you all the time!
2 c many people remember things by seeing them
3 a
4 a
5 c but at first you may not know what is useful, so
   better to write more rather than less
6 b much easier to remember like this, especially if it
   is the same chunk you heard it in c alphabetical
   order is easier to find but less easy to recall
7 c you can't write everything about every word –
   that's the job of a dictionary
8 f though pronunciation is nearly always useful
9 a great, now sell the film rights b okay but not so
   useful professionally speaking c yes yes yes
10 trick question – all the answers are correct!

1.2.b

  O   O   O
radiographer   intravenous   condition
  O   O   O
deteriorate   haemorrhage   department

Alternative key:
radiOGrapher intraVENous   conDItion
deTERiorate   HAEmorrhage dePARTment

1.2.c

        O
1 Please sit down.
        O
2 Have a nice day!
   (shop assistant to customer as they leave a shop)
  O   O
3 Mutton dressed as lamb.
   (a disapproving expression said of a woman who
   wears clothes more suitable for a younger woman)
        O
4 Who's a mucky pup?
   (said affectionately to someone who has got dirty,
   often a child)
        O
5 What did your last servant die of?
   (said jokily to somebody who is
   giving you lots of work to do)

Unit 2

2.2.b

1 B 2 E 3 A 4 D 5 C

Unit 3

3.2.a

A 7 **B** 3 **C** 11 **D** 1 **E** 10 **F** 4 **G** 5 **H** 2 **I** 8 **J** 6 **K** 9

3.4.b Asking your colleagues to help you whilst you admit a patient

a I need to admit Mrs Plymouth, would you be able to look after my other patients in bay 4?

b Do you think you could help me while I admit Mrs Plymouth, my other patients are Miss Coventry and Mr Derby?

c I'm really busy admitting Mrs Plymouth – would you have time to do Mr Derby's obs?

d Could you give me a hand looking after my patients as I'd like to concentrate on admitting Mrs Plymouth?

e I'm finding admitting patients quite time consuming – do you think you could help me out with my other patients?

3.4.c Sample answers

1 Previous medical history and/or surgery
   a Have you been in hospital before?
   What was that for?
   b Do you know why you are in hospital this time?
   Can you tell me why?
   c Are you being treated by a doctor for any illness or condition at the moment? What is the illness or condition?
   d Are you taking any medicines at the moment? Could I see the medicines you have brought with you?

2 Home and family
   a Can you please tell me your address?
   b What type of accommodation do you live in? (house, flat, bedsit, residential home)
   c Who do you live with?
   d Do you have stairs in your accommodation?
   e Do you have family and/or friends locally?
   f Is your home near to shops and public transport?

3.4.c Sample answers (continued)

3 Eating and sleeping routines
   a What do you usually have for breakfast/lunch/evening meal?
   b What foods do you prepare for yourself?
   c Do you have any special preferences or needs such as low fat diet vegetarian etc?
   d What food do you enjoy?
   e Do you usually sleep well at night?
   f Do you need any help getting ready for bed?

Unit 4

4.1.a Suggested answers

OT = occupational therapist
POP = plaster of Paris
OAP = old-age pensioner
pt = patient
A&E = Accident and Emergency
RTA = road traffic accident
r = right (but could be lots of other things, so potentially ambiguous)

4.2.a

1 my mother (r) an father
2 D(y) O(w) A
3 be dan brea(k)fast
4 roa (d) traffi caccident
5 have I (y) ever told you (w) about …?
6 pu tit ona piece o(f) paper

Unit 5

5.1.b Here are some possible answers

1 Lack of evidence-based knowledge
2 Lack of materials or time to research and read
3 Lack of skills or confidence in delivery of facts
4 Lack of time to talk to patients and their relatives
5 Ethical issues
6 Lack of self-awareness
7 Specific values or beliefs
8. Patient not willing or able to participate

5.1.c

1 Working with patients on an analysis of their needs and planning realistic, agreed targets (L, S, W, CA)
2 Selecting information relevant to your patient (R, CA, T)
3 Translating health education information into patient-friendly language if necessary (S, CA)
4 Showing empathy (particularly if patient has not had success in changing habits or lifestyle) (L, S, CA)
5 Respecting your patient's beliefs or values (CA, T)
6 Being aware of learning models i.e. looking at different approaches as well as assessing your patients' preferences (T, R, CA)

5.2.b

/ second cubicle you have Vera Smith / she's a sixty year old under Mr Hartley / she came in with a trimalleolar fracture of the right ankle / she's for a check X-ray today / the form has been signed and taken to the department / she's completed her IV antibiotics / post op observations are stable / there's no neurovascular deficit / windows should be checked tomorrow the fifth of march and the back slabs to be replaced / she's going to be seen by the physio regarding mobility non-weight bearing / she lives in the bungalow with her family and she can go home when safe / and outpatients in two weeks / I have referred this lady to the OT for a general assessment

5.2.c

1 year
2 broken
3 mobilizing
4 medical
5 continent
6 so

5.2.e

a 5 future action already arranged (going to form)
b 4 telling the story (past form)
c 3 recent action (perfect form)
d 1 present fact (is)
e 3 recent action continuing (perfect form + ing)
f 1 present fact (is)
g 1 present fact (has)
h 5 future action (perfect form)
i 3 recent action (perfect form)
j 5 telling the story (past form)

5.3.a

1 **main courses**: a, e, f, h and j
  first courses:b
  sweets: c, d, g and i
2 **traditional British**:b, c, d, f, g, h, j
  multicultural: a, e. i
3 **suitable for vegetarians**: a, b, c, d, g, h, i
  suitable for diabetics: all except e

5.3b

1 True, though
  a some items are left out
  b very few people eat a traditional English breakfast any more, especially at home in the mornings
2 False – most people take it with milk, and sometimes sugar.
3 True
4 True
5 True
6 False, although some people believe you should not drink coffee last thing at night, because it may stop you sleeping

5.3.c

Box 1: sunflower spread; all the others contain milk or cheese products.

Box 2: Hot Sweet; the others all contain vegetables.

Box 3: Fresh Fruit can't be eaten by someone who has chewing problems.

5.3.d

1 N>P
2 P>N *Okay then look for the V symbol next to the item*
3 N>P
4 N>P
5 N>P
6 P>N *Okay. Let's see what we can do about that*
7 P>N
8 Trick question! This is a relative to a nurse.

5.3.e

1 c 2 f 3 a 4 b 5 d 6 g 7 e

5.5.a suggested answers

1   o O o o   O   b
He was **all over the place**.
He didn't know how to behave

2   o o o O   d
In the event the whole meeting was rather disappointing
What actually happened

3   o o O o o O o o   a
For all practical purposes you can work normally.
In the real rather than idealized or theoretical world

4   o   o o O o o o c
Don't even think about it, I said when he wanted to come in for coffee. That is not a good idea.

5.5.b

   o o o o o O o   O

1 I'm just going to do your obs.
   O o o

2 That's it!
   o O o o O o o o O

3 Just pop yourself up on the bed.
   o o O o o o O o o o O

4 Do you want to have a look at your X-ray?
    O   o o o O

5 Come and have a seat.
    O o   o o o o O

6 What we're going to do now….
   o o o o o O o O

7 Do you want to ring your wife?
   o   O o O o o o O o o o O

8 We'll help you shift up the bed in just a minute

5.6.a

a figure 6
b figures 3 and 4
c figures 2 and 5
d figure 1

5.6.b

1 Pakistani
2 twice
3 rate
4 number
5 rose
6 1976
7 rose
8 6
9 decrease
10 and the highest rate

5.6.c

1 increase as a verb is pronounced with the stress on the second syllable: inCREASE.
If it's a noun, the stress is on the first: INcrease (same rule with decrease and record).

5.6.d

1 There was a sharp increase in 1992
2 The number of notifications has declined since 1990.
3 Compared with 2000, 1998 was relatively quiet.

181

Unit 6

6.2.a

Moving a patient to operating theatres on their bed

Transferring a patient from bed to floor, chair to commode or toilet

Moving a patient in bed e.g. if they need to go up the bed

Sitting a patient up in bed

Encouraging or supervising a patient using a banana board, monkey pole

Helping a patient turn onto their side/back

Moving a patient in a wheelchair

6.2.d

a Lack of patient co-operation

b Your patient is lacking in confidence

c You feel your colleagues don't always follow correct moving and handling procedures

d Lack of appropriate equipment

e You have not had training and/or experience in using this equipment

f Not enough colleagues to help you when you need them

g You are not confident enough to do the task alone

h You have hurt your back in the past and are worried about this happening again

6.4.a

1 N 2 N 3 N 4 P 5 P 6 N 7 N
8 both 9 N 10 P

6.5.a

a peacefully

b fearful

c happiness

d happy

e beauty

f encouragement

g constantly

h resentful

i equip

j able

k hopeful

l act

6.5.b

a specialty or specialism

b catheterise

c personally

d society

e imaginatively

f action or activity

g explicit

h to stress or to be stressed

i gently

j improved or improving

k document

l responsibility

m accountable

n infection

6.5.c

Suggested answers:

1 infection 2 specialism 3 improve 4 responsible
5 socialise 6 gentle 7 explained 8 personal 9 active
10 document

6.7.b

Mr Plymouth's been having some trouble sleeping, haven't you Mr. Plymouth?

His observations have been stable for the last 12 hours

Mr Plymouth's apyrexial

His urine output's been improving

He's been mobilising to the bathroom this morning

He's eating and drinking well

Mr. Plymouth's wound's healing nicely

6.7.e

Can Mrs. Kent start taking fluids now?

Can we do anything about the problems with e.g. pain, nausea?

What do you suggest for e.g. this tickly cough, swallowing problems?

Any idea about a potential discharge date?

So you're going to order an ultrasound and change the medication?

So you don't think there's anything we can do about that?

6.7.f

She/he may ask questions (though may need encouragement from the nurse)

The patient may have asked the nurse to ask questions on her/his behalf, e.g. Mr Plymouth was wondering if he could go outside into the garden in the wheelchair?

When the nurse makes her comments she usually includes the patient by using phrases such as 'Is that right, Mr. Plymouth?'

That's what you said isn't it, Mr Plymouth?

When the team depart your patient may want you to recap, summarise and clarify what was said. This may be because they don't understand some of the language

6.7.g The house officer

Mr Kent had a chest X-ray yesterday - it shows a decrease in consolidation of the left lung

Mrs Rose is three days post-op - she's feeling so much better

I've changed Miss Brown's antibiotics and she's apyrexial now

We had a bit of a rough day yesterday but things seem to be much more settled now

You're almost ready to go home now - isn't that right Mrs Page?

6.7.g The physiotherapist

Miss Shrewsbury is doing really well on the stairs

We seem to have shifted some of the consolidation

Mr Kent is working really hard on his exercises

6.7.g The consultant

I think we need to change the antibiotics and do another X-ray in 48 hours

I'd like to see what happens over the next 24 hours and have another look in the morning

We'll take you to theatre tomorrow and try to sort all this out, is that all right with you Miss Brown?

Can we get an ultrasound and blood cultures and make a decision tomorrow?

Can we get some more fluids going in and try sips of water later today as long as there's no further vomiting?

6.7.g The patient

When do you think I'll be able to go home, doctor?

Will I need another operation, doctor?

Will I able to walk properly soon, doctor?

I'm still having a lot of pain, is that normal?

Unit 7

7.2.d

1 No, thanks. I'll ring back later
2 She's with a patient at present
3 It's Paul Green from A&E
4 Thanks very much
5 That's right

Unit 8

8.1.a

Handwashing – to be carried out between patient contacts, after removal of protective clothing and after contact with body fluids and blood, before and after invasive procedures and before handling food

Cuts and Abrasions – Skin with a cut or abrasion should be covered with a waterproof and breathable dressing

Gloves - Non-powdered gloves should be worn for patient care where contact with body fluids is likely. Latex gloves are usually available and alternatives for those with latex allergies. Sterile gloves are necessary for invasive procedures

Needlestick injury - Any needlestick injury should be reported immediately to the nurse in charge. Occupational health should be notified (or Accident and Emergency outside office hours). An incident form should be completed

Waste disposal – Three major groups you will come across. Household waste to go in black bags. Clinical waste e.g. dressings, incontinence pads, colostomy bags to go in yellow bags. Sharps, needles, scalpels etc. to go into a puncture resistant container

Aprons – Single use plastic. Used when there is a chance of splashes on the clothing

Eye protection – Check the policy in your workplace

Spillages/Disinfection – Various types of cloths/mops and solutions according to local policy. Likely to include detergent for general cleaning and Sodium Hypochlorite 0.1% or 1% for disinfection

8.1.b

1 I 2 D 3 F 4 E 5 B 6 C 7 G 8 A 9 H

8.2.a

Hair care

a Shall I get your brush/comb for you?
b Do you need some help combing the back of your hair?
c We'll see if you can get a shower soon so that you can give your hair a wash. What do you think?
d Would you like me to do your hair for you?
e There is a hospital hairdresser. Would you like me to get you an appointment?
f Your hair looks fine but if I get your mirror you might want to check it?

Mouth care

a Shall I get your toothbrush/toothpaste for you?
b Would you like me to clean your teeth/dentures for you?
c What do you usually do with your dentures?
d Would you like me to clean your mouth with these sponges?
e Would you like to rinse out your mouth
f (to patient with low level of consciousness) I'm just going to clean your mouth with sponges and water, OK?

8.3.b

colour yellowy, greenish, dark brown,
consistency watery, mucousy, loose, semi-formed
other comments offensive

8.4.a

my sit-upon **c**   wee-wee **c**   go for a slash **b**
use the washroom **b**   faeces **a**   urinate **a**
number ones **b/c**   stool **a**   piss **b**

8.4.b

Medical and formal: faeces, urinate, commode, sluice, stool
Medical and informal: to pass water, bottle
Non-medical and formal toilet paper
Non-medical and informal: wee-wee, piss, potty, go for a slash, my sit-upon, number ones, loo roll, waterworks, bunged up, wet myself, the runs, use the washroom, have a poo

8.4.c suggested answers only

Patient: Nurse, I need to do a <u>wee </u>

Nurse: OK, Mr Severn, I'll bring you a <u>bottle</u>

Patient: Ta

Nurse: Have you <u>passed water</u> already today?

Patient: No. In fact, I'm a bit worried about it Usually my <u>waterworks</u> are fine, but since I've been in hospital…

Nurse: Oh, don't worry, Mr Severn, it's quite normal

Patient: And the other thing is that when I <u>go for a slash</u>, my, you know, my piss is a bit of a funny colour

Nurse: I see. And when did you first notice this?

Patient: Yesterday evening

Nurse: Well, I'll mention it to the doctor, and we might need an <u>MSU</u>

Patient: A what?

Nurse: Sorry, Mr Severn, that means a midstream urine specimen…

Resources

R.1.a What role a buddy can play?

A peer

A support person

A confidant

Someone who is available to be with you

Someone who is a good listener (listens without judging)

Someone who is willing to explore your experience as well as his / her own thoughts, feelings, behaviour

Not a substitute manager, i.e. not responsible for your actions!

R.1.b What is the value of a buddy system?

It allows you to learn from each other and to give and receive encouragement and support

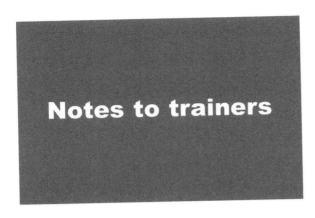

Notes to trainers

A note about the cultural perspective of Hospital English

Hospital English uses the terms 'British' and 'English' to refer to the behaviour of people of the dominant white culture of the UK from London and the south east of the country. In some parts of the wider country the truly multicultural nature of people's lives is abundantly clear. Whilst it is true there is greater recognition now of the diversity of approach needed to serve all sections of our community with dignity and respect, the norms of expected behaviour in professional public life (and levels of expected communication skill) still relate to this dominant culture. This is why there is some emphasis in Hospital English on recognising and relating to these cultural expectations.

However, as you grow more confident in your job, it is up to you to decide how far your own specific cultural and clinical expertise would actually help you in your professional practice where this diverges from standard practice. There are many good reasons for explaining your cultural standpoint at the appropriate time including enhancing your whole team's understanding of diversity.

How this book is organised

There are eight units which provide over three hours structured study each week and many opportunities for reflection and observation in the workplace.

Each unit has four sections:

Language Study looks mainly at issues of pronunciation and intelligibility. It is designed to be used with non-language teachers. In this section we also have designed tasks to encourage the nurses to build up their vocabulary, particularly their colloquial vocabulary and regional or dialect words.

The **Professional Focus** syllabus is intended to be a stimulus only, not comprehensive coverage of these issues. It is ideal if you can invite a visiting speaker from the hospital to give a short talk on the topic and give an up to date perspective of your own hospital procedures. If not, you may be able to get additional material from your library or from nursing journals.

The Scope of Practice section is designed to help the nurses understand their own limitations and work safely within them. They need to understand that their scope will be changing as they develop new professional skills and responsibilities and particularly once they have achieved their registration. The concepts of autonomy and accountability need constant reinforcement as they are often very new to international nurses.

Working with Others is where the communication skill and confidence building activities are located. These tasks should be explored through role plays and practice scenarios as far as possible. Try to get the nurses on their feet and really using the language rather than sitting and talking about it.

> If you want to know more about teaching using practice scenarios and other techniques for workplace-based learning please contact Arakelian Programmes and enquire about our five day trainer development course which runs three times a year.

Exercises, tasks, answer keys and assignments

Tasks and exercises can be completed either in class in pairs or small groups or can be set for homework.

Exercises provide quick practice in aspects of language – normally vocabulary and pronunciation. This course does not have an explicit grammar syllabus so if a nurse is struggling with the rules of the language then you should direct them to a bookshop to buy a good grammar practice book in General English.

Tasks are normally either observation or reflective tasks

Observation tasks need to be carried out while the nurses are at work. They should be encouraged to notice the behaviour and language around them.

Reflective tasks can be carried out in class or as homework. These aim to bring together knowledge and experience so the nurses can deepen in self-awareness and plan their own learning. It is important that emphasis is put on reflecting on incidents where communication was difficult or confusing. It is good to give a few minutes in each lesson to some reflective writing.

Answer keys

Most exercises have an answer key which is located at the end of this section under each Unit. These normally give you suggested answers to most of the tasks. If you are not a trained nurse these should give you adequate language to support the class appropriately.

References

References are written in the text next to the quotation. Most of the books and journals in the references should be available in your medical library.

✎ Assignments

Assignments should be set and adapted to the needs of the individual nurses. Not all topics will be relevant or needed. If the nurses have a heavy burden of clinical learning then it may be appropriate not to set assignments. If they are largely super-numary then each assignment gives some focus to their time.

Because, in our experience, some assignments take longer to produce than others, we recommend the following assignment schedule to trainers over a ten week period.

Feedback on assignments can be in the form of class discussion.

At the end of the course it is good practice to give some one to one tutorial time, possibly using the Assignment 8 as a starting point – to celebrate the individual's progress and to plan their future learning.

Suggested Assignment Timetable

Assignment	Class 1	Class 2	Class 3	Class 4	Class 5	Class 6	Class 7	Class 8	Class 9	Class 10
1 Plan of area	Set	Hand in	Feed-back							
2 Organisation Chart		Set	Hand in	Feed-back						
3 Evaluating Equipment		Set		Hand in	Feed-back					
4 Patient Profile			Set		Hand in	Feed-back				
5 Talk				Set				Talk	Talk	Feed-back
6 Your team						Set			Hand in	Feed-back
7 Transfer Planning						Set			Hand in	Feed-back
8 My Action Plan								Set	Hand in	Feed-back

Communication skills classes proposed outline structure

There are many ways of conducting a three-hour communication skills class depending on the teacher and teaching environment. Taking one unit a week as a basis, negotiate the syllabus with your class and adapt these materials. You may need to jump around the units as necessary. Below is a suggested sequence for a lesson.

For variety and to cover the syllabus most of the following elements should be included most weeks.

1 New lexicon language

Sharing and exploring new vocabulary from My Personal Lexicon or from Hospital English Language Study section.

2 Reflection on socio-cultural adaptation

Looking at collected examples of cultural maps and answering questions about use of English or life outside the hospital.

3 Development of confidence and assertiveness skills

Running practice scenarios based on experiences in the past week recorded in My Professional Identity Notebook or from Hospital English Scope of Practice section.

4 Practical workshop on communication micro-skills

For example, using the telephone, from the Working Together section.

5 Assignments

Setting and clarifying the learning objectives for the assignments, feedback on each assignment and preparation for the next.

6 Tutorials

Individual teaching or feedback from the teacher.

7 Buddy time

The buddy time is for peer-mentoring. Pair up the nurses with their buddies early in the course and they can use some time in class to share experiences while you can take the opportunity to give other nurses' individual support. Otherwise they can conduct the peer-mentoring in their own time and write it up in their Professional Identity Notebooks.

Lecture input is very welcome each week and can support the Professional Focus sections. Invite the specialist in your hospital to come and talk for forty minutes. Allow another twenty minutes for concept checking and vocabulary review.

Suggested marking criteria for assignments

These assignments should be kept in My Brilliant Portfolio as evidence of your learning. See page 166 for more information on portfolios.

Why not give yourself a mark out of 10 for each of the following criteria?

Assignment 1

- Would the plan be of practical use to a new member of staff?
- Does it include relevant detail?
- Is it labelled clearly?
- Does it have a legend or key if needed?
- How much work did you put into the assignment?

Assignment 2

- Would the chart be of practical use to a new member of staff?
- Does it have relevant detail and few or no gaps?
- Does it show the relationships clearly?
- How much work did you put into the assignment?

Assignment 3

- Did you complete the task in the time available?
- Is the equipment and its operation described accurately?
- Did you use a wide range of sources of information?
- Would your guide be useful to a new member of your team?
- How much work did you put into the assignment?

Assignment 4

- Is the profile clear, readable and well-organised?
- Would it be of practical use to another member of staff?
- How much work did you put into the assignment?

Assignment 5

Communication

- How well did you structure your talk with verbal signposts?
- Could your audience follow your talk?

Content

- Did you summarise the main information appropriately?
- Was it relevant and interesting for your audience?

Speaking and listening skills

- How well did you respond to questions?
- How intelligible was your pronunciation?
- How much work did you put into the assignment?

Assignment 6

- Was the questionnaire relevant and well-presented?
- Were the interviews conducted successfully?
- Would the findings be of practical use to another member of staff joining the team?
- How much work did you put into the assignment?

Assignment 7

- How many people did you speak to and involve in your research
- How many sources of information did you find?
- Is your written research clear and well-presented?
- Would your research be of practical use to another member of staff joining the team?
- How much work did you put into the assignment?

Assignment 8

The value in this assignment is in identifying how far you have progressed and what skills you need to work on. Try to find time to talk to your mentor or professional development nurse about your next steps in continuing learning.

- Is the report clear, readable and well-organised?
- Is it of practical use to you (and your manager) in planning your continuing learning?
- How much work did you put into the assignment?

About Arakelian Programmes

Arakelian Programmes Limited was formed by Catharine Arakelian, a former senior lecturer at Oxford Brookes University. Her research into the issues of adult migrant worker education lead to the development of cultural adaptation programmes for nurses. The company now designs highly effective intercultural language and communication skills programmes for international staff and their managers in a variety of sectors, and also trains teachers in the UK and Europe.

Some of our other activities

Communication skills classes for nurses

- We have a team of licensed teaching associates who can deliver classes in Hospital English in your hospital.

Working alongside international nurses

- One day training workshops for practice supervisors and mentors.

Teaching Hospital English and communication skills

- Five day trainer development course for nurse educators and teachers working with international staff in the workplace.

Consultancy

- Design of educational programmes for international nurses wanting to move on from Grade D status.
- Design and delivery of adaptation and induction programmes for NHS hospital trusts.
- International English Language Testing Scheme exam preparation.

Please contact

6, Lakesmere Close

Kidlington

Oxford

OX5 1LG   UK

telephone: 01865 849768 fax: 01865 849769

email: info@arakelian.co.uk www.arakelian.co.uk

Thank you so much for the excellent teaching during the course which helped me to find a job and will help me in my future career.
Vesselka Stoyanova, R.N. successfully moving from Grade D general nursing role to Cardiology nurse in a prestigious teaching hospital.

I was surprised by the teaching method. It was in detail and has developed my confidence and intelligibility. It was brilliant.
Nurse trained in India – Leicester 2002